HYPERACTIVITY
IN
CHILDREN

HYPERACTIVITY IN CHLDREN
Etiology, Measurement, and Treatment Implications

Edited by
Ronald L. Trites, Ph.D.
Head, Neuropsychology Laboratory,
Royal Ottawa Hospital
and
Associate Professor,
Departments of Psychology and Psychiatry
University of Ottawa, Ottawa, Canada

University Park Press
Baltimore

UNIVERSITY PARK PRESS
International Publishers in Science, Medicine, and Education
233 East Redwood Street
Baltimore, Maryland 21202

Typeset by American Graphic Arts Corporation.
Manufactured in the United States of America by
The Maple Press Company.

Proceedings of the Symposium on Hyperactivity in
Children held in February, 1978, Ottawa, Canada.

Library of Congress Cataloging in Publication Data

Main entry under title:

Hyperactivity in children.

    Papers presented at a symposium held in Ottawa,
Canada, Feb. 1978.
    Bibliography: p.
    Includes index.
    1. Hyperactive children—Congresses.   I. Trites,
R. L.
RJ506.H9H97   618.9'28'58   79-1087
ISBN 0-8391-1400-1

Contents

vi   Contents

Contributors

L. Bartley
Child Development Center
Department of Pediatrics
Georgetown University School of
  Medicine
Washington, D.C. 20007

C. Burg, M.A.
Child Development Center
Department of Pediatrics
Georgetown University School of
  Medicine
Washington, D.C. 20007

C. Keith Conners, Ph.D.
Professor of Psychiatry
Program Director, Developmental
  Neurobiology
Western Psychiatric Institute and
  Clinic
University of Pittsburgh
Pittsburgh, Pennsylvania 15261, USA

J. Thomas Dalby
Department of Psychology
University of Calgary
Calgary, Alberta, T2N 1N4, Canada

Virginia I. Douglas
Department of Psychology
McGill University
Montreal, Quebec, H3A 1B1, Canada

H. Bruce Ferguson, Ph.D.
Department of Psychology
Carleton University
Colonel By Drive
Ottawa, Ontario, Canada

Kjell Hole, M.D.
Department of Physiology
University of Bergen
Bergen, Norway

Marcel Kinsbourne, M.D., Ph.D.
Neuropsychology Research Unit
Hospital for Sick Children
555 University Avenue
Toronto, Ontario, Canada

Hallgrim Kløve, Ph.D.
Department of Clinical
  Neuropsychology
Institute of Psychology
University of Bergen
Arstadveien 21
N-5000 Bergen, Norway

Eric J. Mash, Ph.D.
Department of Psychology
University of Calgary
Calgary, Alberta, T2N 1N4, Canada

Bruce A. Pappas, Ph.D.
Department of Psychology
Carleton University
Colonel By Drive
Ottawa, Ontario, Canada

P. O. Quinn, M.D.
Child Development Center
Department of Pediatrics
Georgetown University School of
  Medicine
Washington, D.C. 20007

Judith L. Rapoport, M.D.
Unit on Childhood Mental Illness
Building 10, Room 3N 204
National Institute of Mental Health
Bethesda, Maryland 20014, USA

Robert L. Sprague, Ph.D.
Director, Institute for Child Behavior
  and Development
College of Education
University of Illinois at Urbana
  Champaign
Champaign, Illinois 61820, USA

James M. Swanson, Ph.D.
Neuropsychology Research Unit
Hospital for Sick Children
555 University Avenue
Toronto, Ontario, Canada

Ronald L. Trites, Ph.D.
Head, Neuropsychology Laboratory
Royal Ottawa Hospital
1145 Carling Avenue
Ottawa, Ontario, K1Z 7K4, Canada

Helen Tryphonas, M.Sc.
Food Directorate
Second Floor East
New Research Center, Health &
    Welfare
Ottawa, Ontario, K1A OL2, Canada

Karen C. Wells
University of Pittsburgh
School of Medicine
Pittsburgh, Pennsylvania 15261, USA

Overview

Ronald L. Trites

A great deal of interest in recent years has been focused on the study of hyperactive children. Although many behavioral traits have been ascribed to the hyperactive syndrome, a parsimonious definition of this condition would likely refer to behavior such as restlessness, impulsivity, distractibility, attentional deficiency, and a tendency to seek stimulus (Burks, 1960; Minde, Webb, and Sykes, 1968; Cohen and Douglas, 1972). However, in spite of an increasing recognition of the general behavioral traits characteristic of many hyperactive children, there is not as yet a satisfactory definition of the disorder.

Another major problem, both in the research and treatment of hyperactive children, lies in the confusion over the etiology of the syndrome. Although this syndrome was first described as a sequellae of neurological disease (for example, Ebaugh, 1923; Kahn and Cohen, 1934), it has been well recognized that there is a conspicuous absence of neurological and electroencephalographic signs in many children diagnosed as being hyperactive (Clements and Peters, 1962). Many investigators are now emphasizing the idea that hyperactivity is the final common pathway for a variety of conditions. For example, in addition to the well-described causes of hyperactivity such as perinatal brain damage and asphyxia, the possible genetic factors have been described. It has been demonstrated in animals that high activity levels can be transmitted genetically (Fuller and Thompson, 1960; Cromwell, Beaumeister, and Hawkins, 1963). There is evidence (Wender, 1971; Vandenberg, 1973) of possible corresponding patterns in humans. Among other causes, immunological factors may also be implicated in some children (Tryphonas and Trites, 1979).

It is perhaps unfortunate that some of the first clear descriptions of the hyperactive syndrome were of children who presumably had neurological disease (Ebaugh, 1923; Strauss and Leihtinen, 1947). The tendency has persisted to equate hyperactivity with brain damage or brain dysfunction. However, it has been argued convincingly by many authors (for example, Pond, 1961) that there is no clear causal relationship between brain damage and hyperactivity. For example, many children with cerebral palsy, head injuries, or epilepsy are not hyperactive. It is equally important to stress that many hyperactive children present no evidence from neurological, electroencephalographic, or other related procedures of structural cerebral damage (Knobel, Wolman, and Mason, 1959). Further confusion arises in many reports when hyperactive children are also presumed to have, by definition, a learning disability. Evidence is beginning to emerge (for example, Ferguson and Trites, 1978) that classification of hyperactive children according to presence or absence of signs of brain dysfunction and/or learning disabilities is important in selecting effective treatment.

The importance of defining hyperactivity, determining etiological factors, and rigourously assessing treatment effectiveness is not just a question of semantics and definitions, but has implications for the lives of a great many children. Hyperactivity and related behavioral problems, both in the home and in the school setting, constitute a frequent cause of referral to outpatient clinics, learning clinics, and other specialized programs. However, despite treatments that have been offered (usually stimulant drugs), follow-up studies have shown that the outcome is often poor. There is abundant evidence emerging that hyperactive children are at risk for school failure, psychiatric problems, or other social adjustment problems such as abuse of drugs, including alcohol (Minde et al., 1971; Mendelson, Johnson, and Stewart, 1971; Morrison and Minkoff, 1975; Riddle and Rapoport, 1976; Blouin, Bornstein, and Trites, 1978).

This book represents the proceedings of a Symposium held in Ottawa, Canada, in February of 1978 that focused on the examination of hyperactivity in terms of its prevalence, a discussion of selected etiological factors, and problems in measurement, and that generally had the goal of summarizing important behavioral traits that it is hoped will eventually lead to the development of an operational definition of the disorder. An effort was made by each of the participants to discuss effective measurement techniques that can be applied to assessing the effectiveness of particular treatment strategies. These goals were considered to be particularly timely in view of the above-described confusion and controversy in the literature concerning prevalence, cause, diagnosis, and treatment of hyperactivity in children.

REFERENCES

Blouin, A. G. A., Bornstein, R. A., and Trites, R. L. 1978. Teenage alcohol use among hyperactive children: A five year follow-up study. J. Pediatr. Psychol. In press.

Burks, H. F. 1960. The hyperactive child. Except. Child. 27:18–26.

Clements, S. D., and Peters, J. E. 1962. Minimal brain dysfunction in the school-age child. Arch. Gen. Psychiatry 6:185–197.

Cohen, N. J., and Douglas, V. I. 1972. Characteristics of the orienting response in hyperactive and normal children. Psychophysiology 9:238–245.

Cromwell, R. L., Beaumeister, A., and Hawkins, W. F. 1963. Research in activity level. In N. R. Ellis (ed.), Handbook of Mental Deficiency. McGraw-Hill Book Company, New York.

Ebaugh, F. 1923. Neuropsychiatric sequellae of acute epidemic encephalitis in children. Am. J. Dis. Child. 25:89–97.

Ferguson, H. B., and Trites, R. L. 1978. Predicting the response of hyperactive children to Ritalin: An empirical study. In R. M. Knights and D. J. Bakker (eds.), Treatment of Hyperactive and Learning Disordered Children: Current Research. University Park Press, Baltimore. In press.

Fuller, J. L., and Thompson, W. R. 1960. Behavior Genetics. John Wiley & Sons, Inc., New York.

Kahn, E., and Cohen, L. 1934. Organic driveness—Brain stem syndrome and an experience. N. Engl. J. Med. 210:748–756.

Knobel, M., Wolman, M. A., and Mason, E. 1959. Hyperkinesis and organicity in children. Arch. Gen. Psychiatry 1:310–321.

Mendelson, W., Johnson, N., and Stewart, M. A. 1971. Hyperactive children as teenagers: A follow-up study. J. Nerv. Ment. Dis. 153:273–279.

Minde, K., Lewin, D., Weiss, G., Laviguer, H., Douglas, V. I., and Sykes, E. 1971. The hyperactive child in elementary school: A five year controlled follow-up. Except. Child. 38:215–221.

Minde, K., Webb, G., and Sykes, D. 1968. Studies on the hyperactive child: VI. Prenatal and perinatal factors associated with hyperactivity. Dev. Med. Child Neurol. 10:355–363.

Morrison, J. R., and Minkoff, K. 1975. Explosive personality as a sequal to the hyperactive-child syndrome. Compr. Psychiatry 16:343–348.

Pond, D. A. 1961. Psychiatric aspects of epileptic and brain damaged children. Br. Med. J. 3:1377–1382; 1454–1457.

Riddle, K. D., and Rapoport, J. L. 1976. A two year follow-up of 72 hyperactive boys. J. Nerv. Ment. Dis. 162:126–134.

Strauss, A. A., and Leihtinen, L. E. 1947. Psychopathology and Education of the Brain-injured Child. Grune & Stratton, New York.

Tryphonas, H., and Trites, R. L. 1979. Food allergy in children with hyperactivity, learning disabilities and/or minimal brain dysfunction. Ann. Allergy 42:22–27.

Vandenberg, S. G. 1973. Possible hereditary factors in minimal brain dysfunction. Ann. N.Y. Acad. Sci. 205:223–230.

Wender, P. H. 1971. Minimal Brain Dysfunction in Children. Wiley-Interscience, New York.

Acknowledgments

The Symposium on which this book is based was funded through project #6606-1445-50 from the Contribution and Awards Division, Research Programs Directorate, Health and Welfare Canada. Appreciation is expressed to Mrs. Jean R. Renaud, Head of Technical Secretariat, Health and Welfare Canada, and her staff for the extensive help in making the arrangements for the Symposium. This included not only arranging the excellent facilities, but providing simultaneous translation and making all arrangements for conference participants and delegates. Secretarial assistance was provided by Mrs. Anna Lee Chiprout and Miss Leah Armstrong, and particularly by Mrs. Lyse Blouin, who had the major responsibility. Dianne Thurber was of considerable help as an editorial assistant, along with Mrs. Anne Price in the final stages of completion.

The Symposium sessions were chaired by Dr. Harold C. Grice, Dr. Robert Knights, and Dr. Jovan Simeon. It was fitting that Dr. Grice, Director, Bureau of Chemical Safety, Food Directorate, Health Protection Branch, National Health and Welfare, chaired the opening sessions, since he played an important supportive role in organizing the Symposium.

Finally, it is with deepest appreciation that the contribution of each of the program participants is acknowledged.

Ronald L. Trites

Models of Hyperactivity

Implications for Diagnosis and Treatment

Marcel Kinsbourne
and
James M. Swanson

In many fields of medicine, it is conventional for speakers to say that very little is known about the disease under discussion and that more work should be done. In contrast, so much is known about hyperactivity that the information has become confusing. Before more work is done, some simplifying generalizations are needed. This is the justification for talking about models. The purpose of models is not to state what is the case, but to suggest studies intended to simplify the tangle of our knowledge.

We completely share Dr. Trites' expressed view that, with the present state of knowledge, the question of etiology is only indirectly relevant to the management of hyperactive children. At this time, insofar as we can help these children, it is only through symptomatic treatment. The drug treatments we have are no less symptomatic for hyperactivity than headache pills are for headaches. With regard to measures to change the environment, they are either symptomatic or as yet not completely validated. The time will come when matters of etiology become of practical importance, but etiological models do not as yet have implications for diagnosis and treatment.

ETIOLOGY

There are three views about the origin of hyperactivity: the notions of a deficit, a delay, or a difference (Kinsbourne, 1975). The deficit model was

1

developed from the brain damage model. It states that, because of early brain damage, some children are unable to develop particular skills, and because of this brain-based deficit, they manifest hyperactive behavior. What is the rationale for this view? Early observations of children and adults who had had encephalitis revealed restless, inattentive behavior in the postencephalitic state (Chess, 1969). This behavior pattern was attributed to damage to the brainstem (Kahn and Cohen, 1934). Others (e.g., Strauss and Lehtinen, 1948; Strauss and Kephart, 1955) have observed that obviously brain-damaged children and adults (particularly those with frontal lobe involvement) behaved in ways that are similar to or even indistinguishable from the hyperactive behavior that is seen in those hyperactive children who do not have obvious signs of brain damage. Thus, damage to the brain in certain strategic locations can generate hyperactive behavior.

Nevertheless, it seems highly unlikely that this is how hyperactive behavior is generally generated in most of the 3 to 5% of the school-age population who receive treatment for the disorder (Wender, 1971). The reason, of course, is that most hyperactive children have no history and yield no findings that a neurologist would regard as prima facie evidence of brain damage. In any case, it is unwise to base a diagnosis of congenital brain damage purely on abnormalities in behavioral development (Clements, 1966). It definitely is possible to diagnose acquired brain damage from purely behavioral evidence; neuropsychologists do this with validity all the time. For example, if an adult manifests an aphasia, this behavior is definite evidence of cerebral damage. However, the matter is less clear with respect to the life-long lack of an ability rather than the loss of a previously held skill. The hypothesis that this lack of ability is necessarily due to difficult-to-detect congenital brain damage has not been supported and today not many physicians diagnose congenital brain damage on the basis of behavioral evidence alone (Eisenberg, 1964; Conners, 1970).

However, there may be functional convergence in the behavior resulting from brain damage and that resulting from other causes; therefore, the behavior can then be managed symptomatically in the same way regardless of its origin. For example, the impulsivity of postencephalitic patients can be lessened by stimulant drugs, just as can the impulsivity of hyperactive children who manifest no signs of brain damage. This similarity of response to medication does not mean that hyperactive children are brain damaged in the same way as postencephalitic patients. We should not forget that the means we have available at this time for helping hyperactive children do not depend on etiology. No one has ever shown that pharmacotherapy or any behavioral therapy is more or less effective in relation to the presence or absence of signs of brain damage.

The second model is the delay model (Kinsbourne, 1973). Hyperactive children are said to have a delay in cognitive development with respect to whatever function it is that they are deficient in (Werry, 1968). This model also has some appeal, since in some ways hyperactive children's behavior could be described as immature. Also, the deficit model fits nicely with the widely held notion that some hyperactives recover spontaneously in adolescence: a developmental lag might have been made up and a gap closed at that age. However, there are two serious reservations about this notion.

One reservation is that the developmental lag model does not necessarily differ from the brain damage model. Brain damage can cause developmental delay; in fact, this is one of the main ways in which early brain damage expresses itself (Hebb, 1942). Second, and more importantly, it is not clear that the behavior of hyperactive children is immature. To diagnose a lag in cognition that can legitimately be called a cognitive soft sign in the neurological examination, one must show that the behavior of the child is like the behavior of a normal younger child. However, the behavior patterns of some hyperactive children are clearly abnormal very early (Stewart, 1970; Cantwell, 1975; Juliano and Gentile, 1975); if some patients' parents are to be believed, the children's behavior is abnormal even from birth. Evidence is accumulating that in some cases the symptoms of hyperactivity do not disappear at puberty; rather, the disorder persists and the continuing symptoms, expressed in different but age-appropriate forms, still relate to inattentiveness (Stewart et al., 1966; Menkes, Rowe, and Menkes, 1967; Laufer, 1971; Mendelson, Johnson, and Stewart, 1971; Minde et al., 1971; Weiss et al., 1971; Denhoff, 1973).

The third model is a difference model, which conceptualizes hyperactive behavior as an extreme form of an underlying dimension of behavior. Although there is no one model that covers all cases, we find the difference model the most useful. Human beings differ with regard to a variety of stable personality styles or temperaments (Chess, 1960), based on genetic diversity (Thomas and Chess, 1968). Buss and Plomin (1975) have suggested that four basic temperaments exist: emotionality, activity, sociability, and impulsivity. When a person occupies an extreme position in terms of one of these basic temperaments, his resulting behavior may be maladaptive for much of everyday living. From this point of view, the impulsive behavior of the hyperactive child is not considered qualitatively abnormal, since all of us behave impulsively sometimes. The difference is that the hyperactive individual behaves impulsively more frequently, if not virtually all of the time, and therefore his behavior fits poorly to the adaptive necessities of most situations. The temperamental continuum associated with impulsivity may be considered an attentional one that at one end produces impulsive behavior (failure to concentrate) and at the other end produces overly cautious behavior (maintaining concentration too long). Thus, no dichotomy between hyperactive and normal behavior is assumed. Hyperactivity is not a disease, but rather a matter of degree of concentration that typifies an individual's cognitive style (Douglas, 1972). How far away from the norm a child must be to merit the term "hyperactive" depends not only on his own behavior, but also on what is expected of him by parents, peers, and the rest of society.

Further evidence consistent with the difference model derives from evidence of the heritability of hyperactivity, as shown in cross-fostering (Safer, 1973), twin (Lopez, 1965), and adoptive (Morrison and Stewart, 1973) studies. These studies were designed to reveal genetic components of familial incidence uncontaminated by environmental factors common to the families. When considering cognitive style as a temperament, a number of other thoughts come to mind that have potentially heuristic value. Give a continuum of impulsivity ranging from very readily suspended concentration all the way to unduly maintained concentration, how does it interact with other temperaments? Buss and Plomin (1975) also identified another (orthogonal) temperament that they called activity level. A high activity level per se cannot be regarded as a clinical problem. However, if a child happens to be at the extreme of the impulsivity dimension and also at the extreme of the activity dimension, that combination may be explosive, because he will act out his impulsivity in a vividly overt fashion. A highly impulsive person who has a low activity level may not act out his impulsivity, but rather contain it within his own thought processes. The hypoactive, inattentive child presents with this pattern of behavior. As Bradley (1950), Laufer and Denhoff (1957), and more recently the American Psychiatric Association (1978) have recognized, activity level is not the primary issue. The hyperactivity symptom complex is more accurately described as an impulse disorder (Laufer and Denhoff, 1957) or an attentional disorder, with or without hyperactivity (DSM-III). It is equally clear, however, that a person's activity level can modify the manifestations of the impulse or the attentional disorder.

COGNITIVE BEHAVIOR AND SOCIAL INTERACTION

When hyperactive behavior is considered in the context of the difference model, it can be related to measurements of cognitive variables. It is important to supplement the observers' impressions, however objectively collected, with direct measurement of behavior, because treatments do not always have the same effects on conduct and cognition (Sprague and Sleator, 1977; Swanson and Kinsbourne, 1978a). The ideal approach is to obtain both observational ratings and performance data. In order to obtain performance measures, one has to know which performance to measure. Therefore, one needs a model of the defects of hyperactive children that is sufficiently precise to lend itself to laboratory evaluation. We have considered this problem in detail (Kinsbourne, Swanson, and Herman, 1978; Swanson and Kinsbourne, 1978b), and we present our working model below.

Hyperactive children are often described as being impulsive or distractible, but it is not as simple as it may seem to directly measure this.

Impulsive behavior seems to be an easily perceived characteristic, but distractible behavior is ambiguous. A person may seem distractible because he is impulsive: he may prematurely think one task is finished and therefore move on to another task. Thus, the impulsive individual distracts himself away from the task at hand—stimulus seeking has a part in this. Another type of distractible individual can be regarded as the exact opposite—the overfocused individual who tends to maintain a particular train of thought too long. He does not seek stimulation, but instead is intolerant of it. He can only study away from noise and from people coming and going. Any little noise jangles through his brain and results in a switch in attention from a relevant task or thought to an irrelevant one. This type of individual is distractible in that he is sensitive to irrelevant external stimuli that most people can effectively ignore, but he may have behavioral manifestations similar to the impulsive individual.

Judging a person to be distractible or impulsive, which sounds so specific, can thus leave open a variety of interpretations, so we use the term "concentration" instead. Rather than considering hyperactive children to be distractible or impulsive, we consider them to be children who are quicker than normal to suspend concentration on any one issue and move on to the next. A direct measurement of behavior would thus be one of the concentration span that a hyperactive child exhibits on a given task. We have used a learning task to do this (Dalby et al., 1977), which is discussed in detail later in this chapter.

Of course, one can pursue the question further and ask why hyperactive children suspend concentration sooner than other children. Could it be explained in terms of their susceptibility to reinforcement? In collaboration with us, Freeman (1978) has been able to show a deficit in avoidance learning in these children. Putting together this data with some of the common behavioral descriptions of hyperactive symptomatology (Wender, 1971), one might hazard the guess that these children have behavior patterns not unlike the adult psychopath. They act as if little that happens depends on what they do. For example, the hyperactive adolescent may truly be surprised, after having smashed a window, that someone objects. He may wonder: "Why are the police bugging me? I can't understand it. What is there to be gained by bothering me?" There is a certain naive, innocent incomprehension that suggests an attitude of inconsequentiality in these children—they do not put together the action and the outcome. This may be why successful reinforcement schedules for hyperactive children must be remarkably consistent and salient, as Douglas (Freibergs and Douglas, 1969) has noted. This also fits in with the experiences of people in close contact with these children (parents, childcare workers, teachers, and others) who report that partial reinforcement does not work. However, life is a case of partial reinforcement, if that, so in life the little scraps of reinforcement that we offer just are not enough to control the behavior of these children.

Once one thinks in these terms, one has to admit that biological causes are not necessarily the only causes for inconsequential behavior. There are certainly environmental events that could also produce the behavior patterns just described. Clearly, if a child is raised in a setting in which nothing he does seems to influence what happens to him, then it is likely that an inconsequential behavior pattern could arise that would be hard to distinguish from a similar pattern that has a constitutional basis. Thus, it is difficult to determine whether the behavioral symptoms of hyperactivity are of biological or environmental origin, nor do we know about what might happen when the constitutional bent toward inconsequentiality coincides with the environment that fosters it. However, we must be aware of a possible functional convergence in hyperactive behavior that may not only be due to one of several biological causes, but also to psychological causes. Laufer and Denhoff (1957) long ago recognized the possibility of a convergence of similar behavior patterns that resulted from constitutional and psychological causes when they emphasized the necessity of confirming a diagnosis of hyperactivity by giving a diagnostic drug trial. Their reasoning was that only the children who were hyperactive due to constitutional reasons would respond favorably to stimulant medication.

DIAGNOSTIC TESTS

In further exploring the possibility of a functional convergence of behavior, we used a simple U-shaped performance curve of a type that has been used to describe the behavior of animals (Broadhurst, 1957) and of abnormalities in some clinical groups (Malmo, 1959). We consider the behavioral effect of stimulant drugs to be related to an individual's placement on a continuum of the type we previously discussed, which describes normal as well as deviant behavior even though the physiological effect may be the same for all.

There are clearly two interacting variables that displace an individual from his preferred location on this continuum. One is the nature and amount of the particular drugs given; the other is the nature of the task. If stimulants are given to a person who is impulsive, he is made more reflective. This is important, because our laboratory findings show that, when used appropriately, stimulants do not merely suppress or change the manner of expression of abnormal behavior, but actually normalize behavior. We believe that this occurs when the patient occupies an extreme end of the underlying dimension in the unmedicated state. If a child is hyperactive in the sense of having inadequate concentration, then we consider him to be at one end of the continuum labeled impulsivity. Medication, then, is assumed to displace the child from the extreme and move him into a more normal placement on this dimension of behavior. Normalization of behavior is thus expected. However, if too much medication is given, the child will be pushed past the normal range and out to the other extreme. This is assumed to result in "overfocused" behavior, which produces performance decrements that are as serious as those produced by impulsive behavior. This overfocused behavior pattern is also assumed to occur if even low doses of stimulant medication are given to an individual who occupies the center of the underlying continuum (in an unmedicated state) or to an individual who occupies the opposite extreme end (reflectivity) from the impulsive individual. In these cases, stimulant medication would not be expected to normalize behavior.

Other drugs are expected to have different effects. For example, sedatives have an effect opposite to that of stimulants. They move people from high to low concentration spans, and, in the case of the impulsive person, make impulsivity even more extreme. Laufer and Denhoff (1957) clearly recognized this when they suggested that an adverse response to phenobarbitone was characteristic of hyperactive children.

The nature of the task is the other important variable. The more salient, innovative, exciting, original, new, or rich a task is, the smaller the deficit of the hyperactive child may be and the less his performance may differ from normal performance. Conversely, the more boring, monotonous, continuous, or lengthy in duration a task is, the greater is the performance deficit of the normal individual. We believe that the nature of the task produces these behavior consequences, because the task alters the placement of an individual on the underlying attentional dimension we have described. Some interesting or exciting tasks may reduce impulsivity in hyperactive children, whereas some dull, boring tasks may induce impulsivity in normal children. Given a task that is boring enough and long enough, anyone would be displaced to the extreme end of the impulsivity dimension, and would be expected to respond favorably to stimulants in terms of performance on that task. We also suspect that if a task is exciting enough, anyone would do worse on stimulants in terms of performance on that task.

These points are pertinent to our method of differentiating between what we call "favorable responders" to stimulants and "adverse responders" to stimulants. This is a pragmatic classification that results from the outcome of a diagnostic drug trial, but it has implications beyond that, because it suggests a different brain basis for the deficit of these two kinds of children. However, in order to implement this classification, it is important to find the right task. If the task is too dreary and too lengthy (too much of a "low level" intellectual task), almost every child will show a favorable response to stimulant drugs in terms of performance on that task. Thus, based on the outcome of the diagnostic drug trial, overtreatment of this disorder will occur. We have shown this to be the case with the Continuous Performance Task (CPT). Working with us, Barlow (1977) found that in double-blind drug/placebo trials in which the CPT is used to determine response to stimulant medication, all children referred with symptoms of hyperactivity showed faster reaction times and fewer errors in the drug condition as compared with the placebo condition, even though only 70% of those referred had shown a clinical benefit from stimulant therapy. Thus, the CPT overdiagnoses the favorable response to medication. If this test were used to determine who should and who should not be treated with stimulant medication, a significant number of false positive cases would result. This would be poor clinical practice and would possibly be dangerous to a significant minority of children who would as a result be inappropriately treated with a potentially harmful drug.

LABORATORY EVALUATIONS

We have tried to find a task on which to base this classification of favorable or adverse responder that is just dreary enough and just long enough so as to approximate a classroom situation. The task that has worked best for us is called "paired-associate learning." It has the characteristic that Douglas (personal communication) referred to when she stipulated the kind of paired-associate task hyperactive children would do badly on: one in which there is no natural connection between the stimulus and the response, so that the child has to generate his own imagery or other form of mediation to associate the two.

The materials used in our task consist of a seemingly interminable number of color slides of animals taken at the Metro Toronto Zoo. The child looks at a screen and views a series of slides. First, he is told arbitrarily that each of these animals is housed in one or another of four alternate zoos (the North, South, East, or West Zoo) and that he has to learn this arbitrary association. Next, he is tested on the list of items; after each error he is corrected, and after each correct response he is verbally reinforced. The child is then rehearsed to the point at which he meets a criterion of two perfect recitations of the list.

We begin on the first day of our testing with a familiarization and practice session in which the list size appropriate for a child's ability is determined (in children between the ages of 6 and about 14, learning ability varies considerably across individuals). On the second day we collect data. Each day has two sessions—a morning session and an afternoon session—and different materials (pictures) are used for each test. Our testing is conducted under double-blind procedures. At the beginning of each session (at 8 o'clock and at 12 o'clock), we give the child a capsule that may contain either an active agent (methylphenidate, dextroamphetamine, or pemoline) or a placebo that is visually indistinguishable from the active pill. We then measure the child's performance on the paired-associate learning test in both sessions by counting the number of errors made before the criterion is met. At the end of the testing, the code is broken and we determine whether the child performed better on placebo or on a drug. If he made fewer errors during the placebo session, we consider him to be an adverse responder to drugs. If he made fewer errors during the drug session, we consider him to be a favorable responder.

Our ability to do this testing within a single day depends on the short-acting characteristic of drugs such as methylphenidate or amphetamine. Our initial research established that methylphenidate takes effect within about half an hour, and the effect is virtually over after 4 hours. Another important point is that it does not matter whether it is the first administration ever, or the tenth, or the hundredth; the effects are essentially the same. Effects do not accumulate, and are not permanent. When a treated child is taken off medication, he is as he was before, whether he had 1 day of treatment or a month or a year or several years. (This is a slight overstatement, because a little tolerance often does develop.) Beyond this, we believe that the response of the child to an acute administration of stimulant drug yields a microcosm of how that child will respond in the future. We have documented this by testing children at yearly intervals—the responses of an individual have remained very similar (Dalby et al., 1977).

What is the fine structure of the learning performance of hyperactive children on and off medication? To examine this, we investigated what has been called the total time principle, in which a certain amount of study time is devoted to learning a certain amount of material. For example, if 60 minutes are available to learn 60 Russian words, then one could study each word once for 1 minute, or twice at different times for half a minute, or four times for a quarter of a minute each. Studies of normal adults and children show that it does not matter which of these strategies is adopted—the total amount learned is a function of the total study time, not of how it is partitioned into individual trials.

We have shown that the total time principle does not hold for hyperactive children when they are in an unmedicated state. We gave the paired-associate learning material at 4 seconds per item for six trials each, or 8 seconds per item for three trials, or 12 seconds per item for two trials. In each case, the material was available for 24 seconds. Our hyperactive patients did worse as the trial duration increased. In other words, they failed to take full advantage of the increased learning time per trial when it was offered. They did better with short exposures (4 seconds) given more often, but did not seem to benefit from increase in time. Thus, we believe that the concentration span of our hyperactive patients is less than 8 seconds. On the other hand, we believe that a normal child's concentration span extends beyond 12 seconds, and therefore he can use the total study time in whichever way it is divided—into 4-, 8-, or 12-second blocks.

Even though the total time principle did not hold for our hyperactive patients during a placebo test, we found that when the same patients were given methylphenidate, the total time principle did hold. Not only did our patients learn better overall, but it no longer made a difference whether they were given 4-, 8-, or 12-second exposure durations. In this regard, they were indistinguishable from normal children on this test. This is a vivid illustration of the fact that stimulants used in the right dosage normalize behavior for the period during which they act. Unfortunately, a drug like methylphenidate does not act for very long.

When the effect of a drug on behavior is investigated, it should be possible to show a time-response relationship between drug administration and the relevant behavior. If a particular performance increases in efficiency as the drug is absorbed and then diminishes as the drug is metabolized, then one can be assured that the behavioral effect being measured is produced by the drug. Although this is the easiest and best way to document a drug effect, there seems to be little such information for psychoactive drugs. Keeping in mind that there are enormous individual differences in the response to stimulant drugs, it is unfortunate that we don't have this information. We are, after all, giving these agents for their behavioral effect, so we need to know what is the behavioral response—when does it start, what is its maximum, and when is it over? We cannot answer these questions on the basis of time curves for the persistence of the agent in the blood, because we don't know what concentration in the blood induces a change in behavior. It is first necessary to measure the behaviors themselves.

We gave a series of patients referred with symptoms of hyperactivity either a placebo or an active drug (at various dose levels) and sampled their performance on the learning test at hourly intervals after each administration (Swanson et al., 1978). In agreement with others (e.g., Fish, 1971), we found that, in our sample of children, only two-thirds were favorable responders and one-third were adverse responders to stimulant drugs on our test. Our favorable responders yielded an average time-response curve showing a minimal effect half an hour after administration, a maximum effect between 1 and 2 hours, and virtual cessation of effect after 4 hours. The adverse responders get worse, but show the same time characteristics. Their worst period is between 2 and 3 hours after administration, and they improve again as the drug wears off. These patterns are shown in Figure 1.

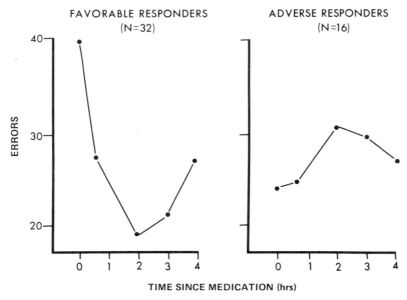

Figure 1.   Time-response curves for favorable and adverse responders.

Consider a group of children who, on single doses of about 10 mg, give clearly favorable responses. Doubling the dosage results in very clear adverse responses. As shown in Figure 2, we can change favorable responders into adverse responders merely by increasing the dose of medication. This shows how crucial it is to give the right dose to ensure optimal response.

Behavioral observations alone may not be sufficient to optimize dose. Consistent with Sprague and Sleator (1977), we have observed that children who are somewhat overdosed may show more acceptable classroom behavior than children who are not (Swanson and Kinsbourne, 1978a). We think that if a child was markedly hyperactive before medication and then is put on what happens to be an overdose of stimulant, the teacher may be so relieved at the fact that he is no longer disrupting the class that the child's slightly glazed and muted, overfocused look is not noticed. Thus, the teacher may rate him as improved when in fact he is in most respects worse off.

Up to this point, we have reported group data, but we have used our diagnostic methods on individual children. For example, a child on 15 mg of amphetamine (Figure 3) who came in to the laboratory was found to act in a mean, uncooperative, and stingy manner (these are subjective observations by observers who were blind with respect to the drug state of the child). As shown in the figure, the patient was initially wild and angry, but a sudden change occurred at about 1½ hours after the drug administration, and he became temporarily generous and considerate. This temporary saintliness wore off within 4 hours, and he then reverted to being loud and incooperative, and running about during testing. Another child, on a placebo initially, began very cooperatively. (The Hospital for Sick Children is very formidable, and even hyperactive children are sometimes temporarily intimidated.) However, this did not last long. Within the hour he was very loud, very active, and bouncing off walls. He then became quiet after being given 5 mg of stimulant medication, and was very attentive. He was still very active and running about, but was at the same time very cooperative. This is important, because it is not the effect of the drug on activity level that is crucial, but the level of attention. In due course, his performance again deteriorated; he was disruptive and again bouncing off walls. A third child (Figure 4) was on placebo initially and was found to be cooperative, but then became active, shouting, and loud. When he was given 10 mg of methylphenidate, he became sullen, uncooperative, very quiet, withdrawn, and angry. At

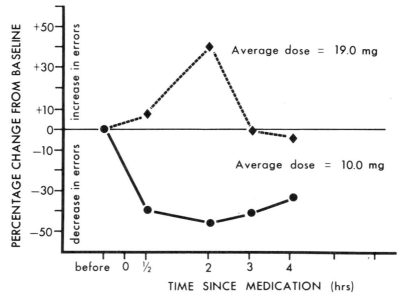

Figure 2.   Effect of increasing dose of medication from 10.0 mg to 19.0 mg.

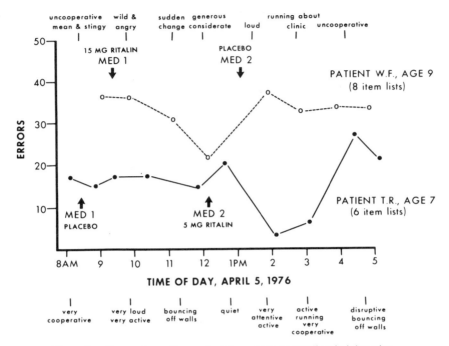

Figure 3.   Comparison of two patients' responses to Ritalin administration.

the same time, his performance on our learning test got worse. We had overdosed him. Fortunately, after 4 hours he was back to his base state, but that sample of behavior has warned us that 10 mg is too much for him.

We have found that some favorable responders do best at 5 mg, some at 10, and some at doses up to 30 or 40 mg. We cannot predetermine which child will need how much of a drug. Five to forty mg is a very wide range of individual difference, and we have found that the optimal dose cannot be worked out even on mg/kg basis. Children who are heavier and older don't need bigger doses; if anything, they need smaller ones. Is this due to differences in the sensitivity of target organs somewhere in the brain, or are these gastrointestinal absorption differences? Perhaps the older children absorb better and therefore achieve effective serum levels with smaller oral doses. We have just developed, in conjunction with Dr. Steven Soldin of the Clinical Chemistry Department of The Hospital for Sick Children, a micromethod for measuring methylphenidate, and we will soon know the answer to that question.

It has been demonstrated in animals and humans that learning while on certain chemical agents is state dependent. If we test for the retention of the learned material or do a relearning experiment, relearning is easier if it is required when the person is in the same state as that in which the material was initially learned. In experiments on adults with alcohol and marijuana, it is well established that what a person learns while on the drug, he relearns better when next on the drug, and what he learns while on placebo, he relearns better when next on placebo. We have reported that the same thing is true of hyperactive children on stimulant drugs (Swanson and Kinsbourne, 1976). On an initial learning day, we had one drug session and one placebo session; thus, material was learned in one state or in the other. On the second day, the children relearned the material of the first day. Again, there were drug sessions and placebo sessions, but in each session, only half of the material that was relearned was material that was presented in the same state as it was initially learned—the other half was presented in the alternate state. As shown in Figure 5, we found that the best learning occurred when initial learning and relearning were accomplished in the same state. Surprisingly, the

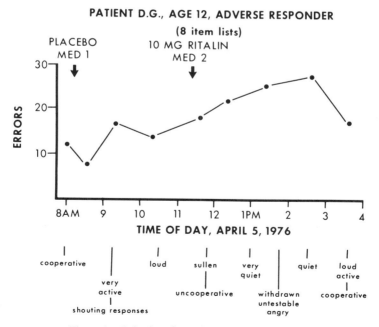

Figure 4.   Behavior of a typical adverse responder.

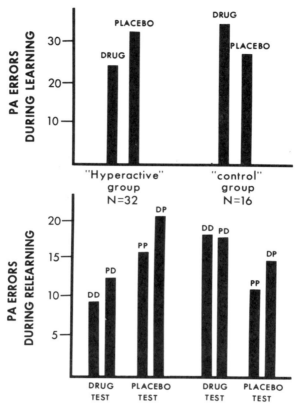

Figure 5. Comparison of paired-associate task behavior under various drug states during learning and relearning.

worst performance was not when learning and relearning occurred in the placebo conditions, but when initial learning was in the drug condition and the relearning was required in the placebo state.

If this also holds for the classroom, our findings are important, because, as a result of the transitory nature of this drug effect, children are "changing states" continually. If a child is on methylphenidate twice a day, which is customary, the effective treatment duration is only about 6 hours in a day. If the drug is used three times a day, the effect may last no longer than 9 hours. We believe that on customary schedules the child receiving medication is functionally "off drug" more of the time than he is "on drug." In the treated child, the level of the drug is constantly changing. It may be that state dependence is associated with different levels of the same drug. If so, it is no wonder that these children, although they seem at the height of the drug effect to be attentive and good learners, haven't retained very much when tested later. This highlights the need for longer-lasting agents. If we are going to use drug management consistently, we need an agent given once a day, the effects of which last for between 16 and 24 hours. We are now investigating several agents, including pemoline, which has quite promising time-response characteristics.

THE DIFFERENCE MODEL OF
HYPERACTIVITY IN RELATION TO BRAIN FUNCTION

The impulsivity dimension of personality has been extensively studied as a component of the characteristic labeled extraversion (Eysenck, 1973). Gray (1967) has pointed out the close similarity of the extraversion-introversion polarity with the Pavlovian polarity of the "strong" versus "weak" nervous system (Nebylitsyn, 1957). The weak nervous system is more sensitive, excitable, and unstable than the strong nervous system. Whereas those with weak nervous systems would tend to avoid stimulation, those with strong nervous systems could be stimulus seekers. On this basis, Eysenck argued that extraverts manifest "stimulus hunger." We could regard hyperactives as extraverts in this respect (Kinsbourne, 1973; King, 1978). At the level of the conceptual nervous system, the possessors of strong nervous systems are spoken of as having high levels of (Pavlovian) cortical inhibition, and at this level Gray (1967) has shown that his strong-weak polarity can be conceptualized in terms of differential levels of activation of the ascending reticular activating system (ARAS). The evidence for diminished arousal in hyperactives (Satterfield and Dawson, 1971; Ferguson and Pappas, this volume; Kløve, this volume) fits well, as does the fact that the stimulant drugs, which by dint of their norepinephrinergic action enhance ARAS activity, diminish the impulsivity and inattentiveness of hyperactive children. The difference formulation of the hyperactive personality thus not only accommodates the known facts about the natural history of hyperactivity, but also provides both a conceptual framework and a possible brain basis for the nature of the disability and its response to psychoactive agents. With regard to the drug effects, these become intelligible when considered in terms of Malmo's (1959) U-shaped relationship between activation and performance, and our experimental studies have documented this in detail.

Individual differences in the level of activation of brainstem mechanisms that control the maintenance of focused attention can, as we have seen, arise as products of genetic diversity. At the same time, it is very likely a person of nonimpulsive genotype can manifest an impulsive phenotype because of brain damage in early development, such that ascending activation is diminished or suppressed. In other words, excitation-inhibition balances, although genetically predetermined, are vulnerable to brain insult, which can change the setting of the balance. Thus, the difference model can accommodate the occasional brain damage origin of hyperactivity as well as its usual occurrence in people for whom acceptable evidence of brain damage does not exist. Like all models, the present model will in time be superseded, but at present it has considerable heuristic value, and it is this that we have attempted to illustrate by studies selected from our research program.

REFERENCES

Barlow, A. 1977. A neuropsychological study of a symptom of minimal brain dysfunction: Distractibility under levels of high and low stimulation. Ph.D. dissertation, University of Toronto, Ontario Institute for Studies in Education.

Bradley, C. 1950. Benzedrine and dexedrine in the treatment of children's behavior disorders. Pediatrics 5:24.

Broadhurst, P. L. 1957. Emotionality and the Yerkes-Dodson Law. J. Exp. Psychol. 54:345–352.

Buss, A. H., and Plomin, R. 1975. A Temperament Theory of Personality Development. John Wiley and Sons, Inc., New York.

Cantwell, D. P. (ed.) 1975. The Hyperactive Child—Diagnosis, Management, Current Research. Spectrum Publications, New York.

Chess, S. 1960. Diagnosis and treatment of the hyperkinetic child. N.Y. State J. Med. 60:2379–2385.

Chess, S. 1969. An Introduction to Child Psychiatry. 2nd ed. Grune & Stratton, New York.

Clements, S. 1966. Minimal brain dysfunction in children. In NINDB Monographs, No. 3. U.S. Public Health Service, Washington, D.C.

Conners, C. K. 1970. Symptom patterns in hyperkinetic, neurotic, and normal children. Child Dev. 41:478–483.

Dalby, T., Kinsbourne, M., Swanson, J. M., and Sobol, M. 1977. Hyperactive children's underuse of learning time: Correction by stimulant treatment. Child Dev. 48:1448–1453.

Denhoff, E. 1973. The natural life history of children with minimal dysfunction. Ann. N.Y. Acad. Sci. 205:188–206.

Douglas, V. I. 1972. Stop, look and listen. The problem of sustained attention and impulse control in hyperactive and normal children. Can. J. Behav. Sci. 4:259–282.

Eisenberg, L. 1964. Behavioral manifestations of cerebral damage in childhood. In H. G. Birch (ed.), Brain Damage in Children: The Biological and Social Aspects. Williams & Wilkins Company, Baltimore.

Eysenck, H. J. 1973. Eysenck on Extraversion. Halsted Press, New York.

Freibergs, V., and Douglas, V. I. 1969. Concept learning in hyperactive and normal children. J. Abnorm. Psychol. 74:388–395.

Fish, B. 1971. The one-child, one-drug myth. Arch. Gen. Psychiatry 25:193.

Freeman, R. 1978. An avoidance learning deficit in hyperactive children. Ph.D. dissertation, University of Waterloo, Psychology Department.

Gray, J. A., 1967. Strength of the nervous system, introversion-extraversion, conditionability and arousal. Behav. Res. Ther. 5:151–170.

Hebb, D. O. 1942. The effect of early and late brain injury upon test scores and the nature of normal adult intelligence. Proc. Am. Philos. Soc. 85:275–292.

Juliano, D. G., and Gentile, J. R. 1975. Will the real hyperactive child please sit down? Problems of diagnosis and remediation. Child Study Monograms 1:1–38.

Kahn, E., and Cohen, L. 1934. Organic drivenness: A brain-stem syndrome and experience. N. Engl. J. Med. 210:748–756.

Kinsbourne, M. 1973. Minimal brain dysfunction as a neurodevelopmental lag. Ann. N.Y. Acad. Sci. 205:263–273.

Kinsbourne, M. 1975. Models of learning disability: Their relevance to remediation. Can. Med. Assoc. J. 113:1066–1068.

Kinsbourne, M., Swanson, J. M., and Herman, D. 1978. Laboratory measurement of hyperactive children's response to stimulant medication. In E. Denhoff and L. Stern (eds.), Hyperactivity. Masson Publishing U.S.A. Inc., New York.

King, C. T. 1978. Hyperactivity, introversion, extraversion and strength of the nervous system in learning disabled children. Ph.D. dissertation, University of Alberta, Edmonton.

Laufer, M. W., 1971. Long term management of some follow-up findings on the use of drugs with minimal cerebral syndromes. J. Learn. Disabil. 4:518–522.

Laufer, M., and Denhoff, E. 1957. Hyperactive behavior symptoms in children. J. Pediatr. 50:463.

Lopez, R. 1965. Hyperactivity in twins. Can. Psychiatr. Assoc. J. 10:421–426.

Malmo, R. B. 1959. Activation: A neuropsychological dimension. Psychol. Rev. 66:367–386.

Mendelson, W., Johnson, J., and Stewart, M. 1971. Hyperactive children as teenagers: A follow-up study. J. Nerv. Ment. Dis. 153:273–279.

Menkes, M. M., Rowe, J. S., and Menkes, J. A. 1967. A 25-year follow-up on the hyperkinetic child with minimal brain dysfunction. Pediatrics 39:398–399.

Minde, K., Lewin, D., Weiss, G., Lavingueur, H., Douglas, V. I., and Sykes, E. 1971. The hyperactive child in elementary school: A five-year controlled follow-up. Except. Child 38:215–221.

Morrison, J., and Stewart, M. 1973. Evidence for polygenetic inheritance in the hyperactive child syndrome. Am. J. Psychiatry 130:791–792.

Nebylitsyn, V. D. 1957. Individual differences in the strength and sensitivity of both visual and auditory analysers. Vopr. Psikhol. 4:153–169. (English translation in O'Connor, N. (ed.) 1961. Recent Soviet Psychology, pp. 52–74. Pergamon Press, Oxford.)

Safer, D. 1973. A familial factor in minimal brain dysfunction. Behav. Genet. 3:175–187.

Satterfield, J. H., and Dawson, M. E. 1971. Electrodermal correlates of hyperactivity in children. Psychophysiology 8:2.

Sprague, R. L. and Sleator, E. K. 1977. Methylphenidate in hyperkinetic children: Differences in dose effects on learning and social behavior. Science 198:1274–1276.

Stewart, M. A., Pitts, F. N., Craig, A. G., and Dieruf, A. 1966. The hyperactive child syndrome. Am. J. Orthopsychiatry 36:861–867.

Stewart, M. A. 1970. Hyperactive children. Sci. Am. 222:94–98.

Strauss, A. A., and Lehtinen, L. E. 1948. Psychopathology and Education of the Brain Injured Child, Vol. 1. Grune & Stratton, New York.

Strauss, A. A., and Kephart, N. C. 1955. Psychopathology and Education of the Brain Injured Child, Vol. 2. Grune & Stratton, New York.

Swanson, J. M., and Kinsbourne, M. 1976. Stimulant-related state-dependent learning in hyperactive children. Science 192:1754.

Swanson, J. M., and Kinsbourne, M. 1978a. Should you use stimulants to treat the hyperactive child? Mod. Med. 46:71–80.

Swanson, J. M., and Kinsbourne, M. 1978b. The cognitive effects of stimulant drugs on hyperactive (inattentive) children. In G. Hale and M. Lewis (eds.), Attention and the Development of Cognitive Skills. Plenum Publishing Corp., New York.

Swanson, J. M., Kinsbourne, M., Roberts, W., and Zucker, K. 1978. A time-response analysis of the effect of stimulant medication on the learning ability of children referred for hyperactivity. Pediatrics 61:21–29.

Thomas, B., and Chess, A. 1968. Temperament and Behavior Disorders in Children. New York University Press, New York.

Weiss, G., Minde, K., Werry, J., Douglas, V. I., and Nemeth, E. 1971. Studies on the hyperactive child. VIII. Five year follow-up. Arch. Gen. Psychiatry 24:409–414.

Wender, P. 1971. Minimal Brain Dysfunction in Children. Wiley Interscience, New York.

Werry, J. S., 1968. The diagnosis, etiology and treatment of hyperactivity in children. In J. Hellmuth (ed.), Learning Disorders, 3. Special Child Publications, Seattle.

Discussion of
"Models of Hyperactivity"

C. Keith Conners

Dr. Kinsbourne's paper fell broadly into two parts. The first was a background description of different models of hyperactivity, and the second presented given methods that would help us to understand the models.

With regard to the models, Dr. Kinsbourne pointed out, correctly, I think, that regardless of which of these etiological models one uses the symptomatic treatment of the child is likely to be the same. He concluded that if one is to behaviorally or pharmacologically treat a child it may not make any difference whether he became hyperactive because of brain damage, through developmental lag, or whatever. I agree with that point of view from a pragmatic and clinical standpoint. However, from a scientific point of view, I think that we really do want to know something about the different ways these children become hyperactive. From the perspectives of ultimately developing preventions as well as developing more targeted treatments that are specific to each child, we need to understand etiology. The treatments for a child suffering from developmental delays could be rather different in some respects from those for a child who has static limitations of the nervous system that aren't going to change. We do not in fact have good differential methods for segregating children with respect to their specific long-term needs.

In the second part of his paper, Dr. Kinsbourne stated that he would provide us with some methods that would help us to understand the first part. These methods, he argues, allow us to learn something about the causes and treatments of the basic disturbances of function. This is probably an overstatement. We have seen some elegant and useful approaches to the measurement of drug effects, certainly a long needed advance. However, I would argue that, just because we understand how the drug works on this particular test, this does not tell us anything about the nature of the underlying defect. The hope here is that, by taking as a model a behavioral test situation where one can control variables such as the time and dosage of the drug, follow the course of the effect, and segregate those who are responding from those who are not, we will then understand something about the nature of the disorder. However, it remains to be established whether or not these results are clinically meaningful and whether they differ for different etiologies or subtypes of children.

Over the years we have done many such tests involving both laboratory and clinical trials. I have always felt that one has to have a combination of clinical observations (of what people actually see the children doing) and laboratory tests in which one can control various parameters, since the two approaches are complementary. So in setting up earlier studies to see what these laboratory tests would predict, we also used paired-associate learning tests. Incidentally, I disproved something that Dr. Kinsbourne said—that there is a difference in the effect of the drug depending on the type or degree of associative learning. We manipulated the degree of associative value on lists to be learned. If you show a picture of a chair and have the word "table" to be associated with it, that is a highly associated item that you would expect to be learned readily on the basis of the association value. If you show the picture of a chair and use the word "mountain," that is a low association. We demonstrated that there was no difference and that drug improves performance on both types of lists. This is because, if you look at other tests that we also gave, they have a strong attentional component and correlate highly with paired-associate learning. When a child is doing a paired-associate learning task, he is not doing a learning task, he is doing an attending task. He is attending to what you are asking him to, more or less. When one intercorrelates a variety of tests, one finds that there is a very strong attentional factor that explains most of the variance.

However, what is more important is that when you try to intercorrelate those laboratory tests with the clinical outcome, the correlations are very, very low. It is very hard to predict how a child will do in the classroom, or in the home, on the basis of his laboratory finding. It is a perfectly reasonable thing to assume that an adverse responder in the laboratory should be an adverse responder at home or at school, but factually this is hard to demonstrate. The reason, I believe, is that the drug effect on the behavior of the child is always a function of the combination of the dosage, the type and degree of the child's CNS defect, and the structure of the environment. This is in fact consistent with what Dr. Kinsbourne has shown in the miniature laboratory experiments—that the structure of the tasks determines what kind of drug effect you get. You can get either an improvement or a worsening by varying the parameters of the tasks. The same is also true in the natural environment. Whether a child responds adversely or favorably to a drug in the natural environment is a function of the structure of that environment. As we heard, the reinforcement contingencies, the classroom structure, and similar things will affect whether or not a particular drug has a particular effect.

If you could coordinate the structure of the environment and the task, and measure both to show that, given a certain degree of structure in the home and a certain degree of performance on the paired-associate learning task, one could predict how the child would behave at home, it would be very useful indeed. However, until you measure the structure in the home or the school, and in effect apply the same kind of analysis to the clinical behavior as you have to the laboratory behavior, there is going to be little relationship. Consequently, I don't really think these will turn out to be very good predictors of performance.

Finally, Dr. Kinsbourne's effort has been focused primarily on a cognitive task. I think that this is a reasonable thing to do, but we have to remember that the cognitive behaviors of the patients are not generally what they have been sent to us for initially. We tend to reinterpret the teachers' and the parents' complaints and say, "Look, your kid does not have a behavior disorder, he has an attentional disorder, and we can explain to you why he behaves funny. It's because his attention system isn't working properly." That is all well and good, except that they know perfectly well that the little bugger gets into trouble all the time and creates disruption, and *that* is what they want to correct. So, presumably you could improve his cognitive skills and not touch his behavioral style, or vice versa. Bob Sprague has posited theoretical curves in which he predicts that a given dose will improve the cognitive function but not the behavioral function. This is entirely consistent with what Dr. Kinsbourne has presented, except that one cannot generalize from one behavior to the other very easily.

In summary, if Dr. Kinsbourne's work is to be useful, he has to demonstrate what has been called "ecologic validity." He should show that his tests predict function in the normal environment of the hyperactive child. He seems to have some suggestive information that the test is reliable enough that one can use it with a given child as a predictor of performance on a moment-to-moment basis. I would like to know what the actual reliability of these scores are for a given child. My own experience has been that the paired-associate tests are just fine for group data, but that they don't work that well with individual children.

Dr. Kinsbourne's work has advanced the level of dialogue in this field and for this we owe him a great debt.

Response to Discussion

Marcel Kinsbourne

Dr. Conners' criticisms of our work fall under two headings: the relevance of basic mechanisms, and ecological validity. With regard to basic mechanisms, we should clearly distinguish practical from research considerations. Much of the confusion in the area of developmental disability has arisen through failure to do this, with the result of injecting speculative and unwanted assumptions into assessments and treatments that are supposed to help children. As practitioners, we are interested in what is known today and not what might be discovered tomorrow. As researchers, our interests are the converse. As I pointed out, at present management is not different for different presumptive etiologies. When research develops methods that are differential in this respect, then etiology would be of practical as well as research interest. I strongly advocate that we do not use in our discussions terminology and concepts that do not directly bear on this management as it may be carried out today.

I would, however, dispute the assertion that our measurements of stimulant response do not contribute to basic understanding of the mechanism of hyperactivity. I think they do. The fact that the drug works is thoroughly revealing because of the way in which it works. Were the drug merely a symptom suppressor or symptom substitutor, then indeed such a nonspecific effect would tell us very little about basic mechanisms. However, as we have shown in experiments such as that with respect to the total time hypothesis, this is not what the stimulants do. Instead, they normalize behavior. Under stimulant, the child's behavior approximates that of normal children. This fact helps us to choose between two alternative neuropsychological models for the deficit.

A neuropsychological deficit may be based on the unavailability of a particular control mechanism (because of either the destruction or the nondevelopment of its brain base), or, it may be due to the relative inhibition of a particular control mechanism, leaving opponent processes in effective control of behavior. Only in the latter case would a psychoactive drug be expected to correct the abnormality, presumably by enhancing the activation of the hitherto insufficiently activated system. Thus, in hyperactivity we do not think that some parts of the brain are functionally absent. Rather, the child deploys with insufficient frequency a facility that he basically does possess. The fact that the stimulants are known to increase transmission at catecholaminergic synapses is consistent with this point of view. We think, then, that some norepinephrinergic or dopaminergic system is rendered normally active by the intervention of the psychoactive agent. It remains to be determined which of the catecholamine systems in the brain is involved in which patients, should it be the case that different ones are involved in different children.

As to ecological validity, we present our methodology as a laboratory procedure contributing to the diagnosis of hyperactivity. Naturally one would not base any such diagnosis totally on this procedure: in clinical medicine it is rarely, if ever, good practice to base a diagnosis on laboratory tests alone. As do Dr. Conners and everyone else, we go through the usual data collection from home, school, and other concerned agencies, the pediatric history and examination, and the interrogation by interview and questionnaire of parents, teachers, and relevant others. Our laboratory procedure is an adjunct source of information: we believe it is an important adjunct.

Incidentally, the test that we use is the one we have in our publications attributed in principle to Dr. Conners, who investigated hyperactivity using the paired-associate technique some years ago. This particular procedure correlates as well with classroom behavior as does any laboratory test of behavior that is known. Of course, the changing situation of the child from moment to moment will affect the issue of whether his response to stimulant is favorable or unfavorable with respect to that situation. Indeed, we have experimental evidence for the concept that an individual's stimulant response is determined by the interaction of his basic constitution, the nature of the drug and dose, the time since dosage of administered drug, and the nature of the task. It is true that, if one prescribes stimulants at any given level, the level cannot possibly accommodate a person's life situation in such a way as to optimize his functioning within the sum total of that range, just as when one prescribes insulin for a diabetic, one has to strike a middle path. After all, no one dose of insulin will accommodate the considerable possible variability of a person's intake of food and output of physical labor. Similarly, we prescribe stimulants in such a way that the child's learning ability will be optimal and clinical reports by parents indicate that this dose is reasonably appropriate for their other activities. Incidentally, the notion (based on Sprague's work) that a much greater dose of stimulant is required to control behavior than to optimize learning is based on fallacious reasoning. We refer to this in some detail in a technical report. In brief, Sprague measured learning ability at a time at which the drug effect was optimal, but measured conduct over longer periods of time, including times when the drug effects were waning or even completely absent. Therefore, it comes as no surprise that in order to obtain the best possible conduct ratings he had to give children high doses (so as to extend the time over which there would be behavioral response). In other words, he was only able to achieve good overall ratings for conduct by substantially overdosing the children, a practice that neither he nor anyone else would in principle encourage.

By no means have we neglected to study conduct as well as cognition: it was only the constraints of time that precluded me from mentioning that aspect of our research program in my talk. We have studied dependent variables such as those yielded by self-concept questionnaires, the Rorschach Ink-Blot Test, and the Children's Aperception Test sufficiently to say that in none of these contexts have we found dose-response requirements substantially different from those that are optimal for learning.

With respect to the question of whether or not our tests are better than other available tools in predicting what the child's drug response will be, the point that 85% of what Dr. Conners terms reasonably selected children will respond to stimulants anyway is not convincing to us. He is referring to those children who score above 15 on both his parent and his teacher inventory. Certainly, if one takes such a conservative sample, we can confirm that virtually all these children will be stimulant responders. However, that conservatism, although useful for research purposes, would do injustice to the average clinic population, since there are a great number of children who score below 15 on one or another questionnaire and yet benefit from stimulant therapy to a substantial extent. This is what our tests are intended to achieve—to separate the adverse from the favorable responders among the children in whom response cannot be predicted with complete assurance by other means. Naturally, the validity of this is ultimately determined by the correlation between the laboratory outcome and outcome in the home and the school. We have much clinical experience with this, and have found the two to relate well in most instances. We are now engaged in formally studying the relationship.

A second thing that our tests do that has never been achieved by questionnaire is to indicate the optimal dose for an individual child. Given that this can vary by a multiple of as much as 10, and given that a mg/kg formula fails utterly to reduce uncertainty, this is a necessary step to take beyond merely identifying a child as a favorable responder.

Prevalence of Hyperactivity in Ottawa, Canada

Ronald L. Trites

Although hyperactivity in children as a clinical entity is frequently diagnosed, the condition is poorly defined, and as yet few prevalence data are available. As a result, pleas have been made (Chalfant and Henderson, 1968) for careful demographic studies 'of hyperactivity in children. This type of study is important for many reasons. First, hyperactivity is perhaps the most frequent cause of referral of children to clinics, special services in schools, and other professional resources. Second, there is increasing awareness that hyperactivity in children is a risk factor for problems in adolescence and adulthood. Data have emerged that suggest that hyperactivity is implicated in delinquency, alcoholism, and other social behavior problems (Blouin, Bornstein, and Trites, 1979).

A case could also be made that hyperactivity may be on the increase. Hyperactivity appears to be the end result of a variety of etiological factors, including prenatal and perinatal complications (Minde, Webb, and Sykes, 1968). With respect to prenatal and perinatal complications, disorders such as marked prematurity or extremely low birth weight, which a few years ago had a high mortality and morbidity, now lead only to a few mild sequellae in affected children, which may include hyperactivity. Since prevalence studies of hyperactivity have not been conducted, there is no conclusive evidence as to whether or not this disorder is actually on the increase. Estimates of the prevalence of the hyperactive syndrome in children vary considerably, ranging from a low

This study was supported primarily by Grant #606-1237-44 from the Research Programs Directorate, Health and Welfare, Canada.

of slightly over 1% up to 15% (Schrag and Divoky, 1975). The most frequently quoted estimates are in the range of 5 to 10%, as cited by Wender (1971). However, the figures do not always relate strictly to hyperactivity, since learning disorders and "minimal brain dysfunction" are also frequently intermixed in the diagnostic groups.

Some authors have suggested that certain professional groups may overestimate the incidence of hyperactivity. For example, Prinz and Loney (1974) concluded that teachers diagnose hyperactivity far more than clinic staff. However, Rubin and Balow (1971) in the Collaborative Perinatal Research Project presented impressive evidence to show that teachers do not seem to overestimate handicaps in children. They show, in their prospective study of 967 children from kindergarten to Grade 3, that 41% (50% of boys and 31% of girls) had school learning or behavior problems. In terms of teacher perceptions of these children, 28% (34% of boys and 22% of girls) were rated by their teachers as having problems in attitudes and behavior, suggesting that teachers do not overestimate problems. To show the range of prevalence estimates within a professional discipline, hyperactivity is diagnosed in 40% of children seen by psychiatrists in the United States (Greenberg and Lipman, 1971), but in only 1.6% of psychiatrically diagnosed children in the Isle of Wight studies (Rutter, Tizard, and Whitmore, 1970).

These large differences are very difficult to account for, but may be due to nothing more than a tendency in other countries to give a different label to the same constellation of behavior traits that we in North America call hyperactivity. Perhaps a difficulty in diagnosis also accounts for the wide variation in prevalence estimates. Unfortunately, no simple diagnostic test of hyperactivity exists. Usually the diagnosis is based on a characteristic behavior pattern that includes traits such as overactivity, restlessness, distractability, and impulsivity. Many attempts have been made to isolate a single, or most important, feature of the hyperactive child. However, taken singly, any of the behaviors commonly associated with the hyperactive syndrome will occur in a very large pro-portion of children. For example, Lapousse and Monk (1958) found that, on the basis of a structured interview with the mothers of 482 children, the prevalence of individual traits was very high. They found, for example, that 57% of the males and 42% of the females were rated by their mothers as overactive, and 27% of males and 26% of females as restless. In a large study of the prevalence of behavior symptoms based on teacher ratings, similar conclusions were reached. Werry and Quay (1971), in a sample of 951 males and 864 females, found that 49% of the males and 27% of the females were rated by their teachers as restless,

36% of males and 20% of females as attention seeking, 46% of males and 22% of females as disruptive, 43% of males and 25% of females as having a short attention span, and 30% of males and 13% of females as overactive. Although the prevalence of individual behaviors in the above two studies, one based on mother ratings and the second on teacher ratings, are not in particularly close agreement, the evidence is rather strong that single behavior symptoms occur with high frequency.

It therefore seems important that, if prevalence studies of hyperactivity are to be comparable, great care should be taken to agree on the exact list of symptoms that are to be subsumed under this syndrome. Also, if the prevalence figures on hyperactivity are to be kept small, the investigators will need to insist either on the presence in each single individual of a large number of behavioral symptoms or that a smaller number are present but to an extreme degree.

THE CONNERS TEACHER RATING SCALE

The study of the prevalence of hyperactivity in a large population obviously demands that a simple, economical, reliable, and valid method of identifying these children be used. Several teacher rating scales have been developed that describe the child in terms of factors such as withdrawal, immaturity, aggressiveness, and overactivity (Patterson, 1964; Quay, 1972; Kupietz and Botti, 1974). One of the most widely used scales is the Conners Teacher Rating Scale (Conners, 1969). This is a 39-item behavior symptom checklist that has five orthogonal factors, four of which are commonly used: conduct problem, inattentive-passive, tension-anxiety, and hyperactivity. The scale has repeatedly proven to be drug sensitive (Werry and Sprague, 1970; Eisenberg and Conners, 1971; Conners, 1972), and has been adopted as part of the battery of tests for drug studies with children published by the Early Clinical Drug Evaluation Unit, Psychopharmacology Research Branch, of the National Institute of Mental Health (United States). The scale had further appeal in that some norms have been developed in various populations, including the midwestern United States (Sprague, Cohen, and Werry, 1974), New York (Kupietz, Bialer, and Winsberg, 1972), and New Zealand (Werry, Sprague, and Cohen, 1975); it has also been translated into French (Trites, 1970). Many studies of hyperactive children use as one of the diagnostic criteria a score of 1.5+ on the Conners scale (Conners, 1972; Sprague and Sleater, 1976).

Each of the items on the Conners Scale is rated by the teacher in one of four categories, including "not at all," "just a little," "pretty much," or "very much." The six items that comprise the hyperactivity rating are:

1. Constantly fidgeting
2. Hums and makes other odd noises
3. Restless or overactive
4. Excitable and impulsive
5. Disturbs other children
6. Teases other children or interferes with their activities

Using a scoring system going from 0 for "not at all" to 3 for "very much," the maximum score is 18. The scores can be converted to a percentage, thus, a mean score of 1.5 on the hyperactivity scale corresponds to a percentage rating of 50.

THE PRESENT STUDY

A study was conducted in the Ottawa, Canada, area in 1976–1977 and 1977–1978 with the aim of obtaining behavior ratings on a large sample of children. The Conners Teacher Rating Scale information, along with additional data described more fully below, was gathered on each child in the study.

Description of Sampling Plan

There are two main school boards in the Ottawa region, the Ottawa Board of Education and the Carleton Board of Education. Both boards are divided into a Public School Board and a Separate (Catholic) School Board, and the latter is further divided into French and English School Boards. Thus, there are a total of six school boards in the Ottawa region and all participated in this prevalence study. A 1-in-4 stratified random sample with proportionate allocation having equal strata was employed. The population of interest was the children from Junior Kindergarten (basically children of age 4) to Grade 6, inclusive, who were residents of the Ottawa-Carleton region during the period from September 1976 through March 1977. From each stratum of four schools (i.e., $N_i = 4$), one school (i.e., $n_i = 1$) was randomly drawn. The sampling frame was organized by locating each school on a map of the Ottawa-Carleton region. Within the jurisdiction of each of the six school boards, a grid was drawn so that each segment (area) of the jurisdictions contained exactly four schools. One school per area (i.e., 1 in 4 schools) was randomly selected. A total of 53 schools were randomly chosen in this manner.

Table 1.   Response rate for the 1977 survey in the
Ottawa-Carleton schools

Disposition	Schools	Classes (All grades)
Responded	51 (96.2%)	589 (94.4%)
No response	2 (3.8%)	35[a] (5.6%)
Total	53 (100%)	624 (100%)

[a] Includes the two schools (with 18 classes) that did not respond.

Response Rate and Sample Characteristics

The sample unit was defined to be the school. Thus, in order to compute the response rate, the school was used as the basic unit. Table 1 shows that 51 of 53 schools completed the necessary information. Thus the response rate was 96.2%. However, it could be argued that if all grades and classes (and hence teachers) within each school did not complete the requisite information, the response rate of 96.2 would be an inflated rate. Accordingly, the number of classes for which total information was given is presented in Table 1. Here, the "response rate" of 94.4% (which includes the 18 classes of the two nonresponding schools) shows that almost all of the teachers in the responding schools completed the requisite information. In fact, only 17 of 606 teachers refused.

Table 2 presents the age distributions of the children in classes from Junior Kindergarten to Grade 6 in the Ottawa-Carleton region. Unfortu-

Table 2.   Descriptive information of sample by age and sex

Age	Males		Females		Total[a]	
	Number	Percentage	Number	Percentage	Number	Percentage
3	30	0.4	17	.2	47	.3
4	463	6.3	421	6.2	885	6.3
5	923	12.6	831	12.3	1755	12.4
6	995	13.7	919	13.6	1916	13.6
7	942	12.9	909	13.4	1853	13.2
8	868	11.9	877	13.0	1745	12.4
9	911	12.5	853	12.6	1764	12.5
10	938	12.8	886	13.1	1824	13.0
11	919	12.6	850	12.6	1770	12.6
12+	317	4.3	206	3.0	524	3.7
Total	7306	100	6769	100	14,083	100

[a] Eight children whose sex was not given and two whose ages were miscoded are included.

nately, we were unable to fully compare these results with the results of the 1971 Canadian Census (Statistics Canada, 1974), since the latter gave age intervals of 0–4, 5–9, and 10–14 years. Similarly, we were unable to compare these results with the true results, since these have not yet become available for use. However, our results showed that, as expected, the percentages of children in each of the ages from 5 to 11 years are fairly constant and that there are approximately as many boys as girls. For the 5–9-year-olds, our results could be compared with those of the 1971 Canadian Census. This comparison showed that the total number of boys in this age range, multiplied by the "blow-up" factor of 4, is 93.7% of the total number of boys in this age range who were attending school in 1971; similarly, the total number of girls aged 5–9 years was 95.0%. In total, our sample yielded 94.3% of the children given as attending school by the 1971 census. It is interesting that: 1) using true 1972 figures, the projections made by the Joint Committee of the school boards for 1975–1976 yielded an overestimate, with the actual attendance being 94.1% of the projected elementary population; and 2) slightly fewer children attended elementary schools in 1975–1976 than in 1971.

In Table 3, the sample distributions by mother tongue are compared with those of the 1971 Canadian Census. From this table, it is evident that the sample yielded only minor discrepancies that can be attributed to the fact that no mother tongue was given for 1.4% of our sample.

Table 4 presents the comparisons between the sample and the population with respect to religion. Our results seemed to slightly underestimate the proportion of Roman Catholics. However, in Ottawa proper (excluding Vanier), our sample proportion of Roman Catholics was 49.1% as compared to 49.2% from the 1971 Canadian Census. Thus, it appears that our sample underestimated the proportions in the Carleton Region. The difference can be explained when it is considered that we measured religion by school attendance. This is not a highly accurate

Table 3. Numbers and percentages of English, French, and others in the Ottawa-Carleton schools survey and in the Canadian Census of 1971

Language	Number in sample	Sample percentage	Number in census	Population percentage
English	9991	70.9	334,110	70.8
French	2552	18.1	97,975	20.8
Other	1339	9.5	39,845	8.4
Unknown	201	1.4		
Total	14,083	100	471,930	100

Table 4.   Numbers and percentages of Roman Catholics and others in the Ottawa-Carleton schools survey and in the Canadian Census of 1971

Religion	Number in sample	Sample percentage	Number in census	Population percentage
Roman Catholic	5530	39.3	222,650	47.2
Other	8553	60.7	249,280	52.8
Total	14,083	100	471,930	100

measure of religious affiliations, since, among other reasons, in rural areas parents may tend to send their children to the nearest school.

In summary, the 1-in-4 sample of the schools in the Ottawa-Carleton region yielded a high response rate and an adequate age and sex distribution, was able to detect the decline in the elementary school population, and produced distributions of language almost identical with the 1971 Canadian Census, and only slightly different proportions of children who are Roman Catholic (the means of measuring religion would explain these slight differences). Sukhatme and Sukhatme (1970) have shown that, when the nonresponse is small (our true nonresponse was less than 4%), its effects on the estimates are negligible.

In addition to completing the 39 items on the Conners Scale, the teachers were instructed to provide additional information on each child: age, sex, mother tongue, estimated learning capacity, actual rate of achievement, language skills, special needs in the classroom (such as remedial reading), and other information. All of the teachers in each of the 53 schools were given personal instruction in the use of the forms, and any questions that they had were answered at that time. At no time was the word "hyperactivity" used; the teachers were merely told that this was a survey of the behavioral characteristics of children in the Ottawa-Carleton region.

For the purposes of individually collecting the work from each teacher and assuring that all ratings were completed satisfactorily, seven graduate students in psychology were employed. In addition to distributing and collecting the teacher ratings, the student research assistants were involved in a validity phase of this study. As a group they received lectures on the hyperactive child both in terms of research findings and clinical description. They also viewed movies of children with learning disabilities and hyperactivity, followed by group discussions on the criteria of hyperactivity. The rating scale was carefully discussed. Each student research assistant then went to two randomly selected classes in each of the seven or eight schools on their list and rated one-third of all children in these classes. The pupils to be rated were randomly selected according to a serpentine procedure beginning with the student in the front of the right hand row, proceeding down row one, up row two, down row three, and so forth. The purpose of this part of the investigation was to see if a trained observer's ratings of hyperactivity would correlate highly with that of the teacher. Inter-rater reliability of the teachers' Conners Scale was checked by having, in all situations in which a child had two or more teachers, each teacher rate the child independently.

RESULTS

Data from the Conners Scale

A total of 14,083 children were rated by their teachers. Using the scoring system of 0–3, the means and standard deviations for the total sample on the four factors of the Conners Scale are presented in Table 5. It can be seen that there are important sex differences on all of the factor scores, with evidence of higher scores by males on all factors except tension-anxiety, for which females obtained higher mean scores.

Most clinical studies using the Conners Rating Scale utilize a 1.5 cut-off on the hyperactivity scale to identify the hyperactive child. If a 1.5 cut-off score on all scales is used, it can be seen from Table 6 that there were slight differences between the Ottawa and Carleton School Boards in the percentages of children who exceeded the 1.5 cut-off point. For example, in the Ottawa Board, which is mainly an urban school board, 15.8% of the children exceeded the 1.5 cut-off rate, as compared with 12.7% of children in the Carleton Board. There was also a higher incidence of conduct problems, inattentive-passivity, and tension-anxiety in the Ottawa Board.

Table 5.   Means and standard deviations for the total sample of males and females on Conners Teacher Rating Scale[a]

	Males		Females		Total sample	
Factor	$\overline{X}$	SD	$\overline{X}$	SD	$\overline{X}$	SD
Conduct problem	0.25	0.44	0.15	0.31	0.20	0.39
Inattentive-passive	0.63	0.66	0.41	0.55	0.52	0.62
Tension-anxiety	0.48	0.53	0.56	0.57	0.52	0.55
Hyperactivity	0.64	0.76	0.31	0.55	0.48	0.69

[a] Means and standard deviations reflect 0–3 scoring scale of factors.

Table 6.   Percentages of children in the Ottawa and Carleton School Boards' jurisdictions obtaining a criterion score[a] on the four factors of the Conners Teacher Rating Scale

Factor	Ottawa School Boards	Carleton School Boards
Conduct problem	3.6	2.2
Inattentive-passive	15.0	12.6
Tension-anxiety	7.6	5.5
Hyperactivity	15.8	12.7

[a] Criterion score is 50% or over.

Utilizing a cut-off score of 1.5 in the total sample, 2.9% of the children were rated as having conduct problems, 13.8% as being inattentive-passive, 6.6% as having tension-anxiety, and 14.3% as being hyperactive. As was expected, there was an approximate ratio of 3 boys to 1 girl with ratings of hyperactivity. The percentage of males and females exceeding the cut-off score on the four factors of the Conners Scale is presented in Table 7. A much larger percentage of males than females received higher ratings on all factors except the tension-anxiety, on which females predominated. The largest sex ratio was on the hyperactivity factor.

In view of the reports in the literature in which the frequency of symptoms tend to decline with age (Werry and Quay, 1971), it was most striking in this study to see the high degree of stability in prevalence ratings across all ages for both sexes on all four factors. For example, with respect to conduct problems it can be seen from Figure 1 that, with the exception of a slight increase for both males and females at age 12, the percentage is extremely stable across the ages. It can be seen from Figure

Table 7.   Percentages of males and females obtaining a criterion score[a] on the factors of the Conners Teacher Rating Scale

Factor	Number			Percentage		
	Male	Female	Total	Male	Female	Total
Conduct problem[b]	298	112	410	4.0	1.7	2.9
Inattentive-passive	1308	636	1946	17.9	9.4	13.8
Tension-anxiety	394	535	929	5.3	7.9	6.6
Hyperactivity	1507	507	2017	20.6	7.5	14.3

[a] Criterion score is 50% or over.

[b] These factors are not mutually exclusive and some children are rated on two or more factors.

2 that there were peaks for ratings of inattentive-passivity at ages 6 and 12, but that at other ages the ratings were very stable for both sexes. With regard to tension-anxiety, seen in Figure 3, females predominated at all ages with the exception of age 4. Although there tended to be slightly more variability among the males, the ratings were again similar. With regard to hyperactivity, it can be seen in Figure 4 that the incidence figures matched those for inattentive-passivity quite closely, with peaks at ages 6 and 12, but again there was considerable stability across ages. (These data, do not, of course, prove that it is the same children across ages who are rated high in each of these groups.) We are currently following up 10% of this sample to assess the stability in individual children of the ratings over ages.

As mentioned earlier, one of the advantages of using the Conners Scale in teacher rating studies is that some normative data have been gathered in other areas. The average scale scores on the four factors of the Conners Scale in the present sample can be compared with those obtained in New Zealand by Werry et al. (1975), in the midwestern

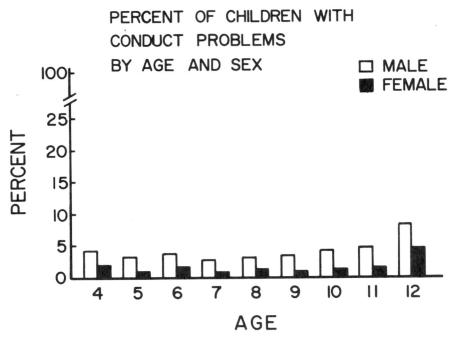

Figure 1.   Percentages of children with "conduct problems" by age and sex.

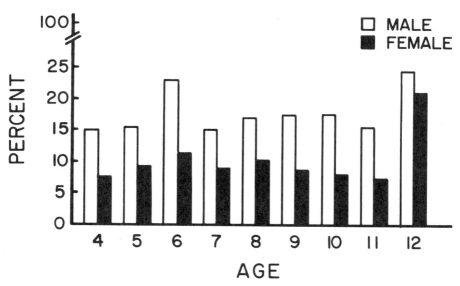

Figure 2.   Percentages of children with "inattentive-passive" behavior by age and sex.

United States by Sprague et al. (1974), and in New York by Kupietz et al. (1972). These comparisons are presented in Table 8. It can be seen that the scores obtained in the present sample match most closely those from the Sprague et al. (1974) study. The similarity in prevalence figures across the four samples gives some confidence that a stage is now being reached such that, if scores on the Conners Teacher Rating Scale are reported in studies being done on children's behavior disorders in different locations, some basis of comparability of the studies can be made. However, the differences between samples are sufficiently large that, as we have pointed out elsewhere (Trites et al., 1978) and as can be seen in Table 9, different cut-off scores need to be employed on the Conners Scale in order to yield roughly equivalent percentages of children who would be identified as hyperactive.

In an attempt to explore different approaches to the analysis of these prevalence data, and with the help of Professor D. R. F. Taylor from the Department of Geography at Carleton University, the data were analyzed by the SYMAP program. This program was developed by Dr. Donald S. Sheppard (1973) of the Laboratory for Computer Graphics at Harvard University. To use this computer program, the coordinates of one or more data points and values associated with them are entered. The program then produces both a contour map and a two-dimensional map. With respect to concentrations of conduct problems in the Ottawa area, it can be seen from the SYMAP represented in Figure 5 that there are definite "peaks" and "valleys," which, it must be stressed, are independent of population density. With respect to ratings of inattentiveness and passivity, it can be seen from Figure 6 that, again, specific areas are implicated. With regard to tension-anxiety, it can be seen from Figure 7 that the same is true.

The SYMAPs in Figures 5–7 were all viewed from the southeast. The program also produced maps from other directions. Figure 8 presents hyperactivity from the northwest view, and Figure 9 presents it from the southwest view. Figure 10 presents hyperactivity from the

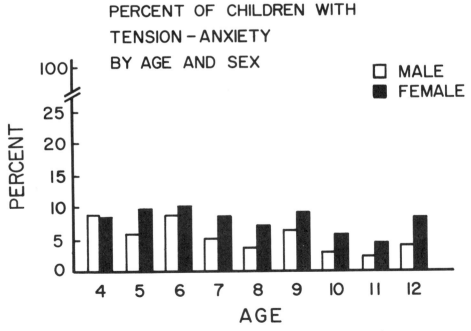

Figure 3.   Percentages of children with "tension-anxiety" by age and sex.

Table 8. A comparison of the norms obtained in New Zealand, the United States, and Canada for the factors on the Conners Teacher Rating Scale

Factor	New Zealand[a] (N = 415)		Midwestern United States[b] (N = 291)		New York[c] (N = 92)		Canada[d] (N = 14,083)	
	$\overline{X}$	SD	$\overline{X}$	SD	$\overline{X}$	SD	$\overline{X}$	SD
Conduct problem								
Boys	1.60	0.53	1.21	0.39			1.25	0.44
Girls	1.42	0.47	1.08	0.30			1.15	0.31
Total	1.51	0.51	1.14	0.35	1.38	0.69	1.20	0.38
Inattentive-passive								
Boys	1.96	0.60	1.60	0.58			1.63	0.66
Girls	1.71	0.58	1.43	0.55			1.40	0.55
Total	1.83	0.60	1.51	0.57	1.82	0.75	1.52	0.62
Tension-anxiety								
Boys	1.61	0.46	1.29	0.33			1.48	0.52
Girls	1.73	0.56	1.35	0.44			1.56	0.56
Total	1.67	0.53	1.32	0.39	1.86	0.62	1.52	0.54
Hyperactivity								
Boys	2.07	0.73	1.56	0.65			1.65	0.76
Girls	1.58	0.65	1.25	0.39			1.30	0.53
Total	1.82	0.78	1.40	0.55	1.75	0.71	1.46	0.68

[a] Werry, Sprague, and Cohen, 1975.

[b] Sprague, Cohen, and Werry, 1974.

[c] Kupietz, Bialer, and Winsberg, 1972.

[d] Trites, this volume. For comparison purposes, the means from the Canadian data have been changed to reflect a 1–4 scoring of items.

southeast view, and it can be seen that the hyperactivity, as well as other behavior problems, tends to occur in particular areas.

SYMAPs can be produced to identify possible differences in patterns of occurrences for boys and girls. Figures 11 and 12 give southeast views of hyperactivity for boys and girls, respectively. It can be seen that there are clear differences in the sex distribution of the ratings, the reasons for which are unclear. We are currently investigating various characteristics of the peaks and valleys to try to understand this further. Such differences in prevalence ratings in the various regions of the city are obvious topics for further research.

Data from Additional Information

Teachers were instructed, in addition to completing the 39-item Conners Scale, to provide information such as how long they have known the

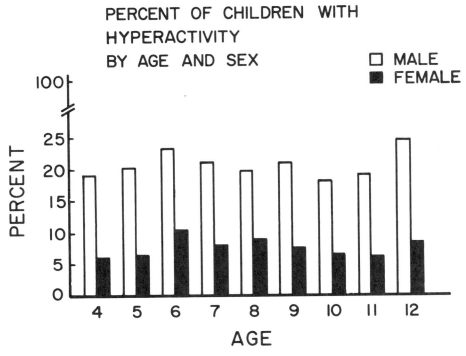

Figure 4.   Percentages of children with "hyperactivity" by age and sex.

Table 9.   Percentages of children identified as hyperactive in four countries according to cut-off score selected on the Conners Scale

Cut-off score	Boys	Girls
1.5 Cut-off		
United States (Sprague, Cohen, and Werry)	9	2
Germany (Sprague, Cohen, and Eichlseder)	12	5
Canada (Trites, Dugas, Lynch, and Ferguson)	21	8
New Zealand (Werry and Hawthorne)	22	9
1.8 Cut-off		
Germany	6	3
Canada	11	4
2.1 Cut-off		
New Zealand	5	4

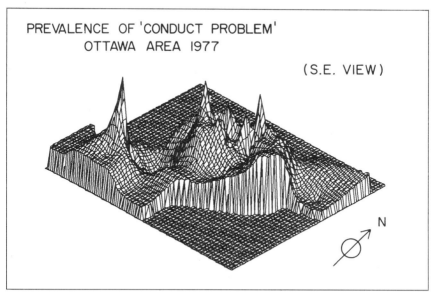

Figure 5.   Prevalence of "conduct problem" in Ottawa area, 1977.

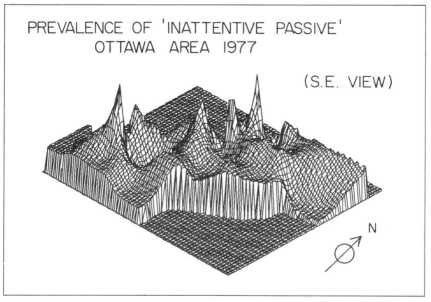

Figure 6.   Prevalence of "inattentive-passive" behavior in Ottawa area, 1977 (SE view).

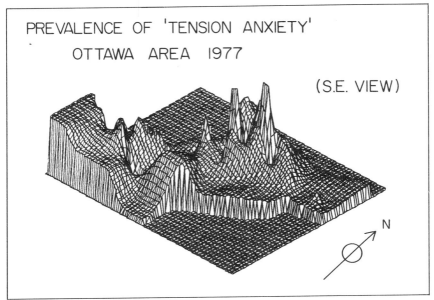

Figure 7.   Prevalence of "tension-anxiety" in Ottawa area, 1977 (SE view).

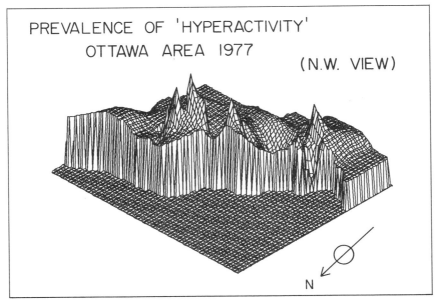

Figure 8.   Prevalence of "hyperactivity" in Ottawa area, 1977 (NW view).

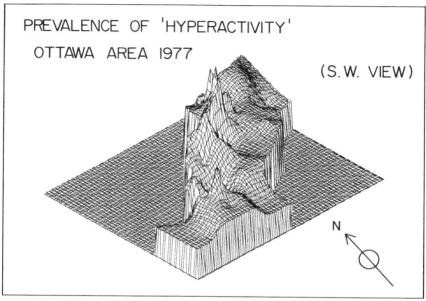

Figure 9.   Prevalence of "hyperactivity" in Ottawa area, 1977 (SW view).

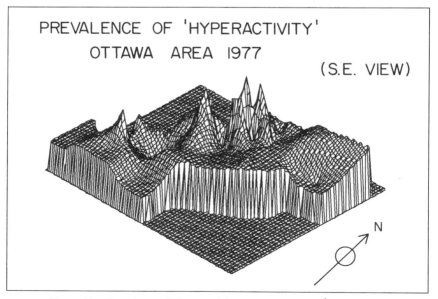

Figure 10.   Prevalence of "hyperactivity" in Ottawa area, 1977 (SE view).

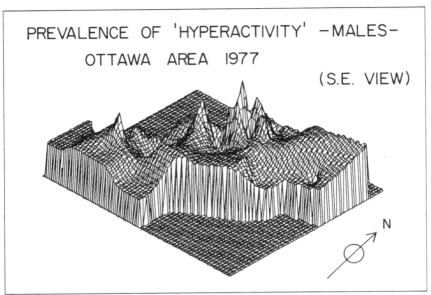

Figure 11.   Prevalence of "hyperactivity" in boys in Ottawa area, 1977 (SE view).

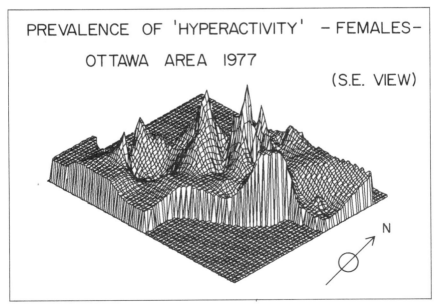

Figure 12.   Prevalence of "hyperactivity" in girls in Ottawa area, 1977 (SE view).

Table 10.   Percentages of children of below average, average, and above average learning capacity obtaining a criterion score[a]

Factor	Below average capacity	Average capacity	Above average capacity
Conduct problem	5.4	3.0	1.6
Inattentive-passive	40.7	12.2	4.0
Tension-anxiety	11.4	6.4	4.7
Hyperactivity	24.3	14.2	9.4

[a] Criterion score is 50% or over.

child and to estimate the child's learning capacity, rate of achievement, language skills, and other factors. Several interesting trends emerged relating this information to the behavior ratings. For example, on the item in which the teacher rated the child according to his learning capacity ("below average," "average," or "above average"), it can be seen from Table 10 that there is generally a reduction, as might be expected, in the prevalence of behavior problems in children as they go up the ability scale. However, it is very important to note that over 9% of children who are rated as above average in learning capacity were also rated by their teachers as hyperactive. The most noticeable change in behavior ratings with increasing ability was for inattentive-passivity, in which over 40% of below average children were rated as inattentive-passive, whereas only 4% of above average children were so rated. When these data were examined by sex (Table 11), the trends were the same for both sexes. However, with respect to hyperactivity, a full 15.6% of boys who were rated by their teachers as above average in capacity were also rated as hyperactive. In terms of actual achievement, as can be seen in Table 12, once again the most noticeable change was on the inattentive-

Table 11.   Percentages of males and females of below average, average, and above average learning capacity obtaining a criterion score[a]

Factor	Below average capacity		Average capacity		Above average capacity	
	M	F	M	F	M	F
Conduct problems	6.6	3.8	4.0	1.8	2.7	0.6
Inattentive-passive	44.8	34.8	15.8	8.1	6.3	1.9
Tension-anxiety	9.2	24.3	5.4	7.5	3.1	6.2
Hyperactivity	31.0	14.6	20.0	7.7	15.6	4.2

[a] Criterion score is 50% or over.

Table 12.   Percentages of males and females of different rates of achievement obtaining a criterion score[a]

Factor	Below average		Average		Above average	
	M	F	M	F	M	F
Conduct problem	8.7	5.5	2.7	1.1	1.5	0.2
Inattentive-passive	43.5	34.7	10.0	5.4	2.6	0.7
Tension-anxiety	7.3	12.4	5.1	7.2	3.5	6.6
Hyperactivity	36.1	17.4	16.5	6.4	9.4	2.9

[a] Criterion score is 50% or over.

passive scale, with 43.5% of boys and 34.7% of girls with below average achievement rated as inattentive-passive, while only 2.6% of boys and 0.7% of girls with above average achievement are rated as inattentive-passive. It is important to note that 9.4% of boys achieving at an above average rate were rated by their teachers as hyperactive. This is less than the 15.6% of boys who were rated as having above average capacity. The difference of 6.2% may represent, in part, the "cost" of being hyperactive. The fact that 9.4% of boys rated as above average in achievement were also rated as hyperactive should act to caution those individuals who tend to equate learning disorders with hyperactivity.

Extensive data have been gathered in this project bearing on the reliability and validity of the Conners Teacher Rating Scale. It was found, for example, that teacher ratings tend to vary somewhat according to the length of time the teacher has known the child. It can be seen from Table 13 that progressively fewer children achieve ratings of hyperactivity and inattentive-passivity over time, whereas ratings of tension-anxiety and conduct problems seem to stabilize in the 1- to 5-month period. In terms of interrater agreement, there were 1154 cases in which two teachers knew the child well. In these cases each teacher rated the child independently. It can be seen from Table 14, in which the

Table 13.   Percentages of children assigned a criterion score[a] relative to duration of contact between child and teacher

Factor	Less than 1 month	1 to 5 months	Over 5 months
Conduct problem	4.0	2.9	2.9
Inattentive-passive	13.4	14.4	12.6
Tension-anxiety	4.3	6.8	6.3
Hyperactivity	15.6	15.0	12.5

[a] Criterion score is 50% or over.

Table 14. Comparison of the Conners Teacher Rating Scales on same children filled out independently by two teachers

Variable	Number of cases	Mean percentage	t-value	df	Two-tailed test
Conduct problem					
1st teacher		5.84			
	1154		-1.12	1153	0.26
2nd teacher		6.24			
Tension-anxiety					
1st teacher		14.37			
	1154		-9.32	1153	0.000
2nd teacher		20.63			
Inattentive-passive					
1st teacher		16.39			
	1154		-1.95	1153	0.05
2nd teacher		17.63			
Hyperactivity					
1st teacher		15.47			
	1154		0.64	1153	0.52
2nd teacher		15.06			

Table 15. Comparison of the Conners Teacher Rating Scale Scores on the same children filled out independently by the teacher and a trained observer

Variable	Number of cases	Mean percentage	t-value	df	Two-tailed test
Conduct problem					
1st teacher		12.24			
	747		6.96	746	0.000
External rater		7.18			
Tension-anxiety					
1st teacher		20.74			
	747		5.26	746	0.000
External rater		16.44			
Inattentive-passive					
1st teacher		25.15			
	747		10.71	746	0.000
External rater		15.03			
Hyperactivity					
1st teacher		25.38			
	747		7.47	746	0.000
External rater		17.75			

percentage scores were compared on the four factors, that the ratings were in high agreement for conduct problem, inattentive-passivity, and hyperactivity. There was, however, a significant difference in the teacher ratings for tension-anxiety. This is a most interesting observation, and may be related to the language background of the child, since there were higher ratings of tension-anxiety among Francophone children as compared with Anglophone children in the sample as a whole. There were, however (Table 15), substantial differences between the ratings of the trained external raters and the teachers on all four factors. Thus, it would appear that trained observers spending only half a day in the classroom do not produce ratings that are in agreement with teacher ratings.

SUMMARY

Data from this study suggest that, in the long term, careful collection of normative data based on sensitive and widely used rating scales such as the Conners Teacher Rating Scale will prove to be of great benefit in arriving at an operational definition of hyperactivity in children. It is hoped that this will, in turn, lead to a resolution of much of the confusion in the research literature as to the prevalence of the disorder, and aid sample selection for treatment studies, thus producing more consistent results.

ACKNOWLEDGMENTS

This study, conducted in conjuction with Bruce Ferguson, Ph.D. (psychologist) and George Lynch, Ph.D. (epidemiologist) is part of a long-term hyperactive treatment program being conducted in the Neuropsychology Laboratory of the Royal Ottawa Hospital. Senior research assistants Barbara Helliwell and Erika Dugas have been largely responsible for data collection and analyses.

REFERENCES

Blouin, A. G. A., Bornstein, R. A., and Trites, R. L. 1978. Teenage alcohol abuse among hyperactive children: A five year follow-up study. J. Pediatr. Psychol. In press.

Chalfant, J. C., and Henderson, R. A. 1968. In G. O. Johnson and H. D. Blank (eds.), Exceptional Children Research Review. The Council for Exceptional Children, Washington, D.C.

Conners, C. K. 1969. A teacher rating scale for use in drug studies with children. Am. J. Psychiatry 126:884–888.

Conners, C. K. 1972. Symposium behavior modification by drugs. Psychological effects of stimulant drugs in children with minimal brain dysfunction. Pediatrics 49:702–708.

Eisenberg, L., and Conners, C. K. 1971. Psychopharmacology in childhood. In N. B. Talbot, J. Kagen, and L. Eisenberg (eds.), Behavior Science and Pediatric Medicine. W. B. Saunders Company, Philadelphia.

Greenberg, L., and Lipman, R. 1971. Pharmacotherapy of hyperactive children: Current practices. Clin. Proc. Child Hosp. D.C. 27:101–105.

Kupietz, A., and Botti, E. 1974. Behavior measurement in pediatric psycho-pharmacology. Am. J. Psychiatry 131:106.

Kupietz, S., Bialer, I., and Winsberg, B. 1972. A behavior rating scale for assessing improvement in behaviorally deviant children. A preliminary investigation. Am. J. Psychiatry 128:1432–1436.

Lapousse, R., and Monk, M. A. 1958. An epidemiologic study of behavior characteristics in children. Am. J. Public Health 48:1134–1144.

Minde, K., Webb, G., and Sykes, D., 1968. Studies on the hyperactive child: V. 1. Prenatal and perinatal factors associated with hyperactivity. Dev. Med. Child Neurol. 10:355–363.

Patterson, G. R. 1964. An application of conditioning techniques to the control of a hyperactive child. In L. P. Ullman and L. Krasner (eds.), Case Studies in Behavior Modification. Rinehart and Winston, New York.

Prinz, R., and Loney, J. 1974. Teacher-rated hyperactive and elementary school girls. An exploratory developmental study. Child Psychiatry Hum. Dev. 4:246–257.

Quay, H. C. 1972. Patterns of aggression, withdrawal and immaturity. In H. C. Quay and J. S. Werry (eds.), Psychopathological Disorder in Childhood, pp. 9–22. John Wiley and Sons, Inc., New York.

Rubin, R., and Balow, B. 1971. Learning and behavior disorders: A longitudinal study. Except. Child. 38:293–299.

Rutter, M., Tizard, J., and Whitmore, K. 1970. Education, Health and Behavior-Psychological and Medical Study of Childhood Development. Wiley-Interscience, New York.

Schrag, P., and Divoky, D. 1975. The Myth of the Hyperactive Child. Pantheon Books, New York.

Sheppard, D. S. 1973. Interpolation in SYMAP Version 4 Contouring Program. Laboratory for Computer Graphics, Harvard University.

Sprague, R. L., Cohen, M. N., and Werry, J. S. 1974. Normative Data on the Conners Teacher Rating Scale and Abbreviated Scale. (Technical Report of the Institute of Child Behavior and Development.) University of Illinois, Champaign, Ill.

Sprague, R. L., and Sleater, E. K. 1976. Drugs and dosages: Implications for learning disabilities. In R. M. Knights and D. J. Bakker (eds.), The Neuropsychology of Learning Disorders—Theoretical Approaches. University Park Press, Baltimore.

Statistics Canada. 1974. 1971 Census of Canada, Ottawa-Hull Census Tract. Catalogue No. 95-745 (CT15B).

Sukhatme, P. V., and Sukhatme, B. V. 1970. Sampling Theory with Applications. 2nd ed. A519 Publishing House, London.

Trites, R. L. 1970. French Translation of Conners' Teacher Symptom Questionnaire. Neuropsychology Laboratory, Royal Ottawa Hospital, Ottawa, Canada.

Trites, R. L., Dugas, E., Lynch, G., and Ferguson, H. B. 1978. Incidence of hyperactivity. Pediatr. Psychol. In press.

Wender, P. 1971. Minimal Brain Dysfunction in Children. Wiley-Interscience, New York.

Werry, J. S., and Quay, H. C. 1971. The prevalence of behavior symptoms in younger elementary school children. Am. J. Orthopsychiatry 41:136–143.

Werry, J. S., and Sprague, R. L. 1970. Hyperactivity. In C. G. Costello (ed.), Symptoms of Psychopathology. John Wiley & Sons, Inc., New York.

Werry, J. S., Sprague, R. L., and Cohen, M. N. 1975. Conners' Teacher Rating Scale for use in drug studies with children: An empirical study. J. Abnorm. Child Psychol. 3:3.

Discussion of "Prevalence of Hyperactivity in Ottawa"

Robert L. Sprague

Dr. Trites is to be sincerely congratulated for undertaking this study involving a very major data collection project from a number of schools, many teachers, and more than 14,000 pupils in Canada. There are continuing controversies about the diagnosis of hyperactivity (Gittelman-Klein, Spitzer, and Cantwell, 1978), and it is my belief that the best way of resolving these conflicts is through empirical data obtained from informed, reliable sources such as teachers. Although teachers are sometimes maligned by radical writers who see the public schools as an oppressive agent of a capitalistic society, it is my firm belief based on years of research in this area that teachers are a unique source of easily available information and that their observations are both reliable and sensitive to experimental manipulations (Sprague and Sleator, 1973; 1977). Following this conviction, we have recently collected similar data from more than 6000 children in three different countries (Sprague, Cohen, and Eichlseder, 1977); these data are referred to in the following discussion of Dr. Trites' paper.

Dr. Trites indicates that there is little or no information from prevalence studies of hyperactivity. There is some important but as yet unpublished work by Lambert and her colleagues at the University of California, Berkeley (Lambert, Sandoval, and Sassone, 1977). She collected samples from public and private schools in the East Bay region of the San Francisco metropolitan area, where 1.7 million people of different ethnic groups and, as is well known, with a variety of life-styles live. Through their sampling process, the authors selected 240 schools and, following negotiation with the administrators of these schools, a sample of 4245 children in grades K through 5 was finally obtained. Lambert used three overlapping definitions of hyperactivity. The definitions are based on who was doing the rating or defining—the child's physician, the child's teacher, or the child's parents. Requiring that all three definers rate the child as hyperactive showed only 1.19% of the population of 4245 children to be defined as hyperactive. This is a figure far lower than many of the scare stories that have appeared in the media (Sprague and Gadow, 1977). Requiring that only the teacher define the child as hyperactive yielded only a 3.3% figure. It is in comparison with these prevalence data, the best that are available at the present time, that Dr. Trites' study should be interpreted.

Dr. Trites cited Rutter's research on the Isle of Wight (Rutter, Tizard, and Whitmore, 1970), which concluded that only 1.6% of psychiatrically diagnosed children were hyperactive. Their interpretation overlooks the behavioral characteristics of the children psychiatrically diagnosed in this study. Quoting from our cross-national study, ". . . a claim has been made based upon interpretation of data from the Isle of Wight that 'only one child in a thousand in England is "hyperactive". . .'" (Stewart, 1976). This is a common interpretation, but, I believe, an erroneous one in view of the data actually presented. In Table 11.1 of the Isle of Wight study, it is reported that only one boy and one girl were diagnosed as hyperkinetic of the total of 82 boys and 44 girls having a psychiatric disorder (Rutter et al., 1970). However, if one looks more closely at the behavior that led to the psychiatric diagnosis, it is clear that the symptomatology that was observed in the boys and girls is very similar to that which is used to diagnose hyperkinesis in the United States. For example, in Table 12.9 of the study the three most common deviant behaviors mentioned are restlessness, fidgetiness, and poor concentration (percentages of boys in the psychiatric group showing these three symptoms are 54.4%, 60.8%, and 81.1% and of girls, 37.5%, 34.9%, and 69.8%) (Sprague et al., 1977). Whether the symptoms of the children are the English symptoms of "poor concentration," "fidgety" and "restlessness" or the American symptoms of ". . . having a short attention span, as being impulsive and distractive, as failing to follow through on instructions and complete work, and as being disorganized and inattentive" (Gittelman-Klein et al., 1978), it seems to me that a rose is still a rose whether it is called a rose or not.

In discussing average ratings on the hyperactivity factor of the Conners' Teacher Rating Scale, Dr. Trites states that ". . . a mean score of 1.5 on the hyperactivity scale corresponds to a percentage rate of 50%." Although this is in fact accurate in the sense that a mean item rating of 1.5 on the six items of the factor (range from 0 to 3 for each item) would give a total score of 9 out of a possible maximum score of 18, I much prefer to discuss mean ratings and percentages on the basis of the population distribution of children rather than item scores represented as percentages of the total score possible. For example, in our initial work obtaining normative data (Sprague, Christensen, and Werry, 1974), we reported for the total sample of normal children a mean item rating of 0.40 for both boys and girls on the hyperactivity factor, with a standard deviation of 0.55. Further, we calculated for the hyperactive group the Z score (hyperactive mean minus normal mean divided by normal standard deviation) for this factor score, and, based on an obtained Z score of 3.22, we suggested a possible cutting score of 1.5 (representing a score 2 standard deviations above the normal mean) as a mean item rating for the six items comprising the hyperactivity factor. Additional studies (Werry, Sprague, and Cohen, 1975; Werry and Hawthorne, 1976) supported these earlier findings.

One of the most interesting aspects of Dr. Trites' study is his attempt to validate teacher ratings against the ratings of student observers who came into the class for a half-day period of time. Such validation attempts are absolutely essential because one needs to know how accurately the teachers can rate their students as compared with independent observers who can closely monitor the ongoing behavior. By using a slightly different scale and ensuring that the teacher and the observers rated the child for the same period of time, Ullman and Barclay (1978) found a high correlation between teacher ratings and independent observations. Using a stringent statistic (Kappa) to assess interobserver agreement, they found that the observers had a mean agreement over four observation categories of $\kappa = 0.81$. More interestingly, however, the observation category of on-task agreed with the teacher rating of on-task at $r = 0.73$, and the observed category of sitting agreed with the teacher rating of out-of-seat at $r = 0.72$, both of which are significant at the 0.01 level.

REFERENCES

Gittelman-Klein, R., Spitzer, R., and Cantwell, D. P. 1978. Diagnostic classifications and psychopharmacological indications. In J. S. Werry (ed.), Pediatric Psychopharmacology—The Use of Behavior Modifying Drugs in Children. Brunner/Mazel, New York.

Lambert, N. M., Sandoval, J. H., and Sassone, D. M. 1977. Multiple prevalence estimates of hyperactivity in school children. In R. Halliday (chair), The Hyperactive Child: Fact, Fiction and Fantasy. Symposium presented at the meeting of the American Psychological Association, August, San Francisco.

Rutter, M., Tizard, J., and Whitmore, K. 1970. Education, Health and Behavior—Psychological and Medical Study of Childhood Development. John Wiley & Sons, Inc., New York.

Sprague, R. L., Christensen, D. E., and Werry, J. S. 1974. Experimental psychology and stimulant drugs. In C. K. Conners (ed.), Clinical Use of Stimulant Drugs in Children. Excerpta Medica, The Hague.

Sprague, R. L., Cohen, M. N., and Eichlseder, W. 1977. Are there hyperactive children in Europe and the South Pacific? In R. Halliday (chair), The Hyperactive Child: Fact, Fiction and Fantasy. Symposium presented at the meeting of the American Psychological Association, August, San Francisco.

Sprague, R. L., and Gadow, K. 1977. The role of the teacher in drug treatment. In J. J. Bosco and S. S. Robin (eds.), The Hyperactive Child and Stimulant Drugs. University of Chicago Press, Chicago.

Sprague, R. L., and Sleator, E. K. 1973. Effects of psychopharmacologic agents on learning disorders. Pediatr. Clin. North Am. 20:719–735.

Sprague, R. L., and Sleator, E. K. 1977. Methylphenidate in hyperkinetic children: Differences in dose effects on learning and social behavior. Science 198:1274–1276.

Stewart, M. A. 1976. Is hyperactivity abnormal? and other unanswered questions. School Rev. 85:31–42.

Ullman, R., and Barclay, C. R. 1978. How accurate are teacher ratings when compared to direct behavioral observations? Unpublished manuscript, University of Illinois.

Werry, J. S., Sprague, R. L., and Cohen, M. N. 1975. Conners' Teacher Rating Scale for use in drug studies with children—An empirical study. J. Abnorm. Child Psychol. 3:217–229.

Werry, J. S., and Hawthorne, D. 1976. Conners' Teacher Questionnaire—Norms and validity. Aust. N.Z. J. Psychiatry 10:257–262.

Discussion of "Prevalence of Hyperactivity in Ottawa"

C. Keith Conners

I would first like to compliment the investigators for a truly amazing job. I am just sorry I didn't obtain a copyright on my scale. Unfortunately, this is one of those things I did in an afternoon, a number of years ago, not thinking that some day some pioneer would like to collect data on 15,000 children.

I think the study is so clearly presented that it hardly bears comment from the point of view of the technique. I think it is a very worthwhile endeavor. It now complements the data that Bob Sprague collected last year in Germany on 5000 German school children (Sprague, Cohen, and Eichlseder, 1977). There is also a study that has recently been completed in Berkeley, California by Nadine Lambert and her colleagues (Lambert, Sandoval, and Sassone, 1977). When you put all these data together they seem to give a remarkably similar picture. The prevalence figures for a disorder will naturally be arbitrary, depending on the cut-off criterion one employs.

You could use 2.5 standard deviations, or some other formal criterion score, as was done here. We don't want to be in the position of the American senator who was alarmed on finding out that half of the American population is below average in I.Q. It's sometimes troubling to people to discover that 50% of the children in a survey are alleged to be above average in activity level. This is what happened in the Lapousse and Monk study (1958). There are epidemiologic studies in which you go to households and knock on the door and say "Is your child overactive?" The mother says, "Compared to what?" and you say, "Compared to the kid next door." "Oh! yes he is," the mother responds, and so it is not surprising that half of the kids are described as being more active than the other half. That type of information has very little actual relevance to our purposes as clinicians and scientists. I think it is pretty clear that if you take the present approach what you are going to end up looking at are the extremes of the distribution. Even assuming that this is the extreme of a normal trait, and that it is not due to brain damage or other abnormality, we should be able to identify those children whose characteristics are extreme enough that their behavior is maladaptive.

I think the next step (and I'm sure these researchers have this in mind) is to see what can be done in the way of selecting out those extreme groups and finding out what other background characteristics, history features, perinatal features, etc. characterize them. And, with a sample like this one, you can really ask that question very skillfully.

One other approach that can be taken with these data is to determine differences among children who have various combinations of the symptoms that make up the general factor of "hyperactivity." One should find that there will be a certain number of kids who have only one of these symptoms. There will be a distribution of those scores and then there will be a certain number who have two of those symptoms, three, four, and so on, in all possible combinations. For six symptoms, there will be six factorial combinations of symptoms, and one could then identify groups that have various combinations of symptoms. Unless these symptoms are merely synonyms for each other, one might be able to differentiate kids who are impulsive but not inattentive, impulsive and inattentive, etc., and begin to see whether these form distinctive clinical groups that are particularly maladaptive or are responsive to particular treatments.

This kind of work forms the background of what we need to know in order to make our clinical work reasonable. When the Isle of Wight study (Rutter, Tizard, and Whitmore, 1970) shows only one or two children who are hyperactive, that is clearly not because there were few hyperactives in England but because the English call what we call hyperactivity something else and those children are placed in a different category.

I met an English psychiatrist once at a symposium in Denmark, and I asked him about the low incidence of hyperactivity reported in English schools. He said he had always thought that hyperactivity was an American disease, but then, as he began to get a few patients in, he became more convinced of it, because every time he would get a hyperactive patient, it would turn out to be the son of an American Air Force pilot living in England, and he seemed to believe it was something we exported. Perhaps it's the American life-style, or television, but I suspect it is a matter of how the children are referred.

I would just like to compliment the investigators. This is a very nice job and I appreciate having my name replicated 13,000 or 14,000 times, even without any royalties.

REFERENCES

Lambert, N. M., Sandoval, J. H., and Sassone, D. M. 1977. Multiple prevalence estimates of hyperactivity in school children. In R. Halliday (chair), The Hyperactive Child: Fact, Fiction and Fantasy. Symposium presented at the meeting of the American Psychological Association, San Francisco.
Lapousse, R., and Monk, M. A. 1958. An epidemiologic study of behavior characteristics in children. Am. J. Public Health 48:1134–1144.
Rutter, M., Tizard, J., and Whitmore, K. 1970. Education, Health and Behavior—Psychological and Medical Study of Childhood Development. John Wiley & Sons, Inc., New York.
Sprague, R. L., Cohen, M. N., and Eichlseder, W. 1977. Are there hyperactive children in Europe and the South Pacific? In R. Halliday (chair), The Hyperactive Child: Fact, Fiction and Fantasy. Symposium presented at the meeting of the American Psychological Association, August, San Francisco.

Evaluation of Psychophysiological, Neurochemical, and Animal Models of Hyperactivity

H. Bruce Ferguson
and
Bruce A. Pappas

PSYCHOPHYSIOLOGICAL MODELS

It is appropriate to begin a review such as this by briefly considering important caveats regarding assumptions and definitions. Constructing neurophysiological models to explain hyperactivity reflects a historic bias, that of assuming some underlying "organicity" to explain the behavior of hyperactive children. Indeed, such modeling often has implied the more tenuous assumption that the same underlying neurophysiological mechanism(s) may account for the behavior of all hyperactive children, despite the impressive array of proposed alternative etiologies (genetic transmission, prenatal and perinatal trauma, lead poisoning, maternal smoking during pregnancy, maturational lag, ingestion of food additives, allergies to foods, and abnormalities of glucose tolerance). Although it seems that the first of these assumptions retains widespread acceptance, the current fate of the latter is unclear. Furthermore, in this review we equate the terms "hyperactive," "hyperkinetic," and "minimal brain dysfunction" (MBD), although we admit that these labels as applied do not entail a complete overlap of symptoms. Even though the distinctions between designations are vague, there does seem to be general consensus that the major symptoms of the "typical" child are the same regardless of the label used.

The past two decades of research in physiological psychology and psychopharmacology offer some elegant examples of the complexities of uncovering the neuroanatomical and/or neurochemical systems underlying simple behaviors in the rat. If we were to review carefully the history of even one such attempt, we would certainly conclude that, at the present time, there is indeed little hope of our being able to discover the brain dysfunction(s) responsible for the variable set of subtle human behaviors that have been designated as childhood "hyperactivity." This search is made more difficult by our disagreement about exactly what behaviors define "hyperactivity" and our agreement that, whatever "hyperactivity" may be, it probably represents the final common pathway for a wide variety of possible etiologies. In addition to these already imposing problems of definition, the fact that our subjects are children limits us to only the most indirect of neuroscience research techniques.

Despite such a pessimistic research prospectus, it is interesting to note that researchers have been proposing brain models or mechanisms to explain hyperactivity for 20 years. These proposals have been varied in the extent to which specific neurophysiological mechanisms are outlined. Yet most models possess the common feature of assuming that, whatever the actual mechanism(s) involved, the result of the dysfunction is some abnormality in the arousal level or arousal function(s) of the central nervous system (CNS). Proposals of problems in CNS arousal are attractive for two reasons: 1) in theoretical terms at least, deviant arousal levels can readily explain the attentional deficits and deviant motor activity by which "hyperactive" children are typified; and 2) the widespread success of stimulant drugs (Millichap, 1973) in treating hyperactivity can be understood in terms of their effects on the catecholamines (Snyder and Meyerhoff, 1973), dopamine, and norepinephrine. These putative neurotransmitters in turn appear to be intimately related to CNS arousal level (Wender, 1976). It is perhaps worth noting in passing that in order to explain a behavioral syndrome that has been attacked as badly defined (Sroufe, 1975; Safer and Allen, 1976; Schuckit, Petrich, and Chiles, 1978) we have invoked a combination of two of psychology's most ambiguous and controversial constructs: arousal and attention. As we shall see, this situation has not made progress impossible, but the area certainly has had its share of methodological and interpretational problems.

There is little to be gained from a systematic review of the many proposed models. In general, the "neurophysiologizing" is loose and the relationships between brain structure and psychological function are vaguely defined. An overview of the area is presented in Table 1, which cross-classifies models according to site and nature of dysfunction. Some of the categorizations are forced (e.g., Clements and Peters, who perhaps should be included in overarousal as well), while others are ubiquitous (e.g., Dykman et al.). They propose a deficit in an attentional-switching mechanism in the diencephalon that allows sensory stimuli to flood the cortex while a deficit in patterned inhibition from the cortex results in an inability to sustain attention. Wender (1976) has adopted a "wait and see" attitude on the arousal question. The general flavor of the modeling can be obtained by examining single examples of overarousal and underarousal models.

Laufer, Denhoff, and Solomons (1957) suggested that the diencephalon acts to pattern, route, and give "valence" to incoming sensory stimuli. They speculated that injury or dysfunction of diencephalic struc-

Table 1. Cross-classification of hyperactivity models according to site and nature of dysfunction

Nature of dysfunction	Site of dysfunction		
	Cortical	Subcortical	Not specified
Overarousal	Dykman et al. (1971) Buckley (1972)	Kahn and Cohen (1934) Laufer, Denhoff, and Solomons (1957) Wender (1976)	Freibergs and Douglas (1969)
Under-arousal	Bradley (1937) Dykman et al. (1972)	Stewart (1970) Werry and Sprague (1970) Satterfield et al. (1974)	
Inhibitory deficit	Knobel, Wolman, and Mason (1959) Clements and Peters (1962) Dykman et al. (1971)	Satterfield et al. (1974)	Shetty (1971b) Conners (1976)

tures would alter resistance at synapses. This unspecific "altered resistance" allows impulses to spread out of usual pathways and irradiate large cortical areas. Thus, subcortical dysfunction results in cortical overarousal, which in turn produces the hyperkinetic behavior syndrome.

Satterfield, Cantwell, and Satterfield (1974) hypothesized that a subgroup of hyperactive children have low CNS arousal and insufficient CNS inhibition. They speculate that both arousal and inhibitory functions originate in the reticular formation. Thus, low arousal and insufficient inhibitory control over motor outflow and sensory input results in the hyperactive child being "driven from within and from without by stimuli that would be ignored by the normal child."

Consideration of these two proposals indicates emphatically that hypotheses about the location and nature of brain dysfunction are ill-defined. Furthermore, the empirical evidence gathered thus far regarding hyperactivity provides no firm basis for tracing any dysfunction to specific brain structures. On the other hand, there is a sufficient data base to allow us to address the question of whether hyperactivity results from overarousal or underarousal of the CNS. The underarousal hypothesis is especially attractive: it has allowed us to use the familiar inverted U function relating performance to arousal (Malmo, 1959) to explain the "paradoxical" improvement in hyperactive children treated with stimulant medication. Data presented recently by Rapoport et al. (1978) extend and support the finding of Shetty (1971a) indicating that stimulant drugs produce the same changes in normal subjects and thus these are not "paradoxical" effects. Nevertheless, if a majority of hyperactive children are hypoaroused in terms of CNS activity, then there exists a dissociation between central and behavioral arousal. Thus, the question of over- versus underarousal is an important issue.

The behavior of hyperactive children, particularly their impairment on psychological tests (e.g., attention), can be interpreted as resulting from either hypo- or hyperarousal of the CNS. Thus, the behavioral data by itself affords us no clue to the central arousal state of these children. Any resolution to the over- versus underarousal question can be accomplished only by using psychophysiological techniques. Most of the relevant literature has recorded peripheral autonomic measures from which the arousal state of the CNS can be inferred (Duffy, 1962). Recent research reports show an increasing number of attempts to monitor nervous system activity directly by recording electroencephalograms and analyzing power spectra and averaged evoked responses to discrete sensory stimuli.

Peripheral Autonomic Indices of Arousal

Electrodermal Measures   In a study carried out to test the overarousal hypothesis, Satterfield and Dawson (1971) reported that "hyperkinetic children" had lower basal skin conductance levels (SCLs), fewer and smaller nonspecific galvanic skin responses (GSRs), and smaller GSRs to nonsignal tones than matched normal controls. When hyperkinetics were retested after administration of a stimulant drug (*d*-amphetamine or methylphenidate) basal SCL increased and spontaneous activity increased, but specific GSRs showed no change. These results prompted the authors, and subsequently others, to postulate CNS underarousal as the underlying cause of hyperactivity. Unfortunately, a review of studies using electrodermal measures reveals that this finding of lowered basal levels has been replicated only once (Kløve and Bu, 1976), whereas a number of studies have reported no differences between hyperactives and controls (Boydstun et al., 1968; Cohen and Douglas, 1972; Satterfield et al., 1972; Spring et al., 1974; Firestone and Douglas, 1975; Zahn et al., 1975; Montagu, 1975; Ferguson, Simpson, and Trites, 1976). The finding of fewer and smaller nonspecific GSRs has not been replicated by studies reporting these measures (Spring et al., 1974; Zahn et al., 1975; Barkley and Jackson, 1977). Investigations of mean amplitude of GSRs to nonsignal stimuli also provide conflicting results; two studies found smaller GSRs for hyperactives (Spring et al., 1974; Zahn et al., 1975), whereas others report no difference between groups (Cohen and Douglas, 1972; Ferguson et al., 1976). Ferguson et al. did report that good responders to methylphenidate showed lower amplitude orienting responses to the first few nonsignal tones than poor drug responders. Finally, Spring et al. (1974) and Kløve and Bu (1976) both report faster habituation of specific GSRs to tones for hyperactives, whereas Conners (1976) found just the reverse and the data of Ferguson et al. (1976) showed no difference. Thus, it is obvious that up to this point in time no single measure has provided clear and reliable evidence from electrodermal measures that hyperactive children suffer from a deficit in basal arousal level or responsivity to nonsignal stimuli.

A number of studies have compared electrodermal responses while hyperactive and control subjects were engaged in a task. During performance of a reaction-time task, normal controls have been found to show increased tonic skin conductance (Cohen and Douglas, 1972; Firestone and Douglas, 1975), increased frequencies of specific GSR responses to reaction stimuli (Firestone and Douglas, 1975; Zahn et al.,

1975), and larger amplitude specific GSR responses (Cohen and Douglas, 1972; Zahn et al., 1975) relative to hyperactives. None of these differences was replicated by Ferguson et al. (1976). Conners (1976) reported that hyperkinetics showed higher conductance than normals when required to withhold a response. Thus, even though these data are not unanimous, they suggest that hyperactives do show lower arousal than controls under on-task conditions.

The effects of stimulant drugs on electrodermal indices of arousal have been examined extensively. Satterfield and Dawson (1971) reported that stimulants (d-amphetamine and methylphenidate) did not increase resting conductance and had no effect on mean amplitude of specific GSR responses, but increased mean amplitude of nonspecific responses. In contrast, Cohen, Douglas, and Morgenstern (1971) found that methylphenidate increased resting conductance but had no effect on mean amplitude of specific responses or frequency of nonspecific responses. Spring et al. (1974), on the other hand, indicated that the only effect of methylphenidate was to increase the frequency of nonspecific responses. Finally, the most comprehensive study (Zahn et al., 1975) showed that medication (d-amphetamine and methylphenidate) produced increased basal skin conductance, decreased mean amplitude of spontaneous responses, decreased specific responses to nonsignal tones, and smaller responses to reaction time stimuli. Most of these drug effects were reduced or disappeared when reanalyzed with basal skin conductance and skin temperature as multiple covariates. It is important to note that, apart from basal skin conductance, these changes in electrodermal measures indicate lower arousal levels on medication. The hyperactive subjects of Kløve and Bu (1976), after treatment with methylphenidate, showed increased basal conductance and decreased rates of habituation of GSR responses to tone. Although the results are again inconsistent across studies, it is important to note that each investigation found that stimulants increased at least one measure of arousal.

Cardiovascular Measures   Resting or tonic heart rate has failed to discriminate between hyperactives and controls (Zahn et al., 1975; Ferguson et al., 1976; Barkley and Jackson, 1977), although Porges et al. (1975) reported that mean base-level heart rate for a subgroup of their hyperactive children was lower than published age norms. Conflicting findings have been obtained for heart rate deceleration responses to nonsignal tones: one study has reported smaller orienting responses for hyperactives (Zahn et al., 1975) and another has found no difference (Ferguson et al., 1976). In addition, several reports (Sroufe et al., 1973; Porges et al., 1975) show that hyperactives have reduced anticipatory heart rate decelerations during the fixed foreperiods of reaction-time tasks, whereas others revealed no difference between these children and controls on this measure (Zahn et al., 1975; Ferguson et al., 1976).

Stimulant drugs have produced variable effects on basal cardiac measures as well. Increased resting heart rates while on medication have been reported in several instances (pemoline, Knights and Viets, 1975; methylphenidate, Barkley and Jackson, 1977), whereas no change has been reported by others (methylphenidate, Knights and Hinton, 1969; methylphenidate, Zahn et al., 1975; d-amphetamine, Zahn et al., 1975). Cardiovascular responses to stimulation have been investigated under drug and placebo conditions. Two independent groups of investigators have reported that heart rate deceleration during the foreperiod of a reaction-time task has increased on methylphenidate (Sroufe et al., 1973; Porges et al., 1975). This change represents a "normalization" of the autonomic response and has been interpreted as an indicator of improved sustained attention. In both cases, the "normalization" of the autonomic response was accompanied by faster reaction-time performance. Unfortunately, Zahn et al. (1975), comparing on-drug and off-drug conditions, found smaller heart rate decelerations but faster reaction times in the off-drug state. In addition, it has been demonstrated that hyperactives' finger pulse volume responses to tones habituate slowly and that treatment with d-amphetamine increases the rate of habituation (Conners and Rothschild, 1973; Conners, 1976).

Overall, the results from cardiovascular measures are similar to those for electrodermal measures. There is evidence that hyperactive children are centrally underaroused and that stimulants "normalize" this underlying deficit. In a most impressive study, Zahn et al. (1975) found MBD children "underaroused" as compared to normals on a wide variety of electrodermal and cardiovascular measures recorded both on- and off-task, and that stimulant medication changed MBD in the direction of normals for basal measures but not for variables generally correlated with attention. Moreover, on virtually every independent variable recorded, there are an equal number of reports finding no difference between hyperactives and controls. Thus, at the present time a conclusion that the behaviors of hyperactive children result from less-than-optimal arousal of the CNS must be made only with caution.

Central Indices of Arousal

Clinical Studies of Electroencephalograph Records   Numerous studies have carried out clinical electroencephalographic (EEG) examinations of children with learning and/or behavior problems. Although the children were not always selected or labeled as "hyperactive," a recurring finding in these EEG screening investigations has been an association of excessive slow EEG activity and hyperactivity (Stevens, Kuldip, and Milstein, 1968; Wikler, Dixon, and Parker, 1970; Hughes and Myklebust, 1971). Those few reports focusing on hyperactive children also have noted a high incidence of this same abnormality (Capute, Niedermeyer, and Richardson, 1968; Knights and Hinton, 1969; Satterfield et al., 1972; Satterfield, Cantwell, Saul, and Yusin, 1974; Grunewald-Zuberbier, Grunewald, and Rasche, 1975). Although the proportion of children exhibiting excessive slowing is not large, it has been interpreted as indicating low CNS arousal (Satterfield et al., 1972; Satterfield, Cantwell, and Satterfield, 1974). Shetty (1971a) found that hyperactive children showing a good clinical response to stimulant treatment (d-amphetamine or methylphenidate) tended to show an increase in resting EEG alpha-activity after intravenous injection of the drug. Poor responders tended to show no change, as did those hyperactives given saline injections. All six normal controls (age not noted) manifested increased alpha-activity after stimulant injection. This increase in alpha-activity following stimulant injection has been interpreted by Shetty (1971b) as reflecting increased central inhibitory capacity—i.e., a good drug response is produced by increased inhibition rather than increased arousal. On the other hand, Knights and Hinton (1969) observed that abnormal EEG records (mostly increased slow activity) were reduced by approximatley 30% on methylphenidate. Also, Satterfield et al. (1972) reported that poor responders to methylphenidate showed increased slow-wave EEG power (0–8 Hz), whereas good responders showed no change on medication. Thus neither of the latter studies provide support for the view that the behavioral improvement due to stimulant treatment reflects increased central inhibition.

Responses to Photic Stimulation Laufer, Denhoff, and Solomons (1957) determined the threshold dose of pentylenetetrazol necessary to cause EEG spike-wave bursts following stroboscopic stimulation. They found lower thresholds in the hyperactive group and that thresholds were raised by administration of d-amphetamine. Shetty (1971b) reported photic driving responses in only 11 of 36 hyperactive children, whereas all six young adult controls showed such responses. Stimulant injection (d-amphetamine or methylphenidate) decreased the incidence of driving responses in hyperactives but left controls unaltered. In contrast, Milstein and Small (1974) reported no difference between minimal brain damaged children and normal controls. Furthermore, a stimulant medication (magnesium pemoline) produced "persistent though nonsignificant" increases in the photic driving score.

Thus, the data on EEG response to photic stimulation provide support for over- (Laufer et al., 1957) and underarousal (Shetty, 1971b) hypotheses, or for no difference between hyperactives and controls (Milstein and Small, 1974). At the same time, the demonstrated effects of stimulant medication include both inhibiting (Laufer et al., 1957; Shetty, 1971b) and arousing (Milstein and Small, 1974) functions.

Averaged Cortical Evoked Responses Buchsbaum and Wender (1973) reported a detailed study of sensory evoked responses in MBD and normal children. Children with MBD had larger amplitude, shorter latency visual evoked potentials, and more variable auditory evoked potentials than normal children. The effects of amphetamine differed for clinical responders and nonresponders: the amplitude–stimulus intensity function decreased in slope for responders but increased in slope for nonresponders. Grouping children according to drug response and analyzing predrug measures showed tha older responders did not manifest the decrease in latency with increasing stimulus intensity that was typical of older normals and nonresponders.

Earlier reports involving evoked potentials are difficult to compare. Satterfield et al. (1972) presented data on auditory evoked responses for responder, nonresponder (to methylphenidate), and control groups. Their analyses contrasted responder and nonresponder groups, but it appears that the hyperactive children may have had smaller responses. Treatment with methylphenidate resulted in amplitude decreases for responders and increases for nonresponders. Conners (1972) found that both magnesium pemoline and d-amphetamine increased the amplitude of sensory evoked responses. Comparing hyperactive children on d-amphetamine versus placebo, Saletu et al. (1975) reported that visual evoked potentials showed increased latencies and a tendency to augment amplitude in the stimulant conditions. The conflicting results of these initial studies are difficult to interpret with regard to the over- versus underarousal hypothesis. More recent investigations have not resolved the problem.

Hall et al. (1976) recorded evoked potentials to four stimulus intensities under conditions of attention and inattention. They found no differences in stability, amplitude, or latency between hyperactive and control children. In addition, they failed to find any relationship between degree of abnormality of evoked potential responding and predrug behavior or drug response. Thus, their data represent a complete failure to replicate Buchsbaum and Wender (1973).

Prichep, Sutton, and Hakerem (1976) recorded evoked potentials under conditions of low and high attention. In the high attention condition, all components of the response from P186-N377 were less positive in hyperactive than normal children. This difference was interpreted as indicating an attentional deficit and lower CNS arousal in the hyperactives. Treatment with methylphenidate tended to "normalize" this deviation.

Halliday et al. (1976) reported two evoked potential measures that consistently discriminated responders from nonresponders to methylphenidate. When shifting from a task requiring active attention to one of passive observation, variability of evoked potentials increased in responders but decreased in nonresponders. From placebo to methylphenidate conditions the amplitude of the N140-P190 component increased for responders. This component has been related to selective attention, and Halliday et al. suggest it represents a deficit that is normalized by methylphenidate.

In summary, the evoked potential literature does not provide entirely consistent results regarding the over- versus underarousal question. The meaning of the obtained differences between hyperactive and comparison children is problematical. Although some data can be interpreted as support for the low arousal hypothesis (Buchsbaum and Wender, 1973; Prichep et al., 1976), this must be tempered by the failure of other investigators to detect any difference between hyperactives and controls. Furthermore, the interpretation of this literature is made more difficult by the possibility that at the present time there may be no way to dissociate the effects of arousal and attention on evoked potential responding (Picton et al., 1978). Yet another source of conflict has been discovered in an interesting article by Satterfield and Braley (1977). From a developmental study of auditory evoked potentials in hyperactive and normal children, they found that younger (7–8 years) and older (10–12 years) hyperactives differed from normals, and that these differences were manifested in distinct components of the evoked potential. There were no differences between groups for children 8–9 years of age. Thus, future research in the area must attend to these important interactions of age and evoked potential differences.

Underarousal versus Overarousal: Summary and Conclusions
Despite the large number of investigations carried out and the wide variety of measures used, we can make no certain conclusion regarding the arousal state of the CNS of hyperactive children. We are faced with conflicting findings from studies examining both peripheral and central indices of arousal. There are a number of easy scapegoats for this failure to find reliable differences on any single index of arousal. First, careful scrutiny would allow us to fault almost every study on one or another methodological point: such specifics as electrode placement, electrode

jelly, interstimulus intervals, stimulus intensity, instructions, and details of data analysis provide fertile ground for questioning individual studies. Alternatively, we could appeal to the obvious heterogeneity of subject populations used. Subjects in the studies cited have been labeled variously as "learning disabled," "minimal brain damaged," "minimal brain dysfunction," "hyperkinetic," and "hyperactive." In earlier studies the more objective inventories were seldom used to quantify behavior, and screening for brain damage, emotional and psychiatric problems, and low intelligence was not always adequate. However, the failure of consistently replicable differences to emerge has persisted throughout a decade that has seen increased standardization of methodology and refinement of subject selection. It is clear at this point in time that, although the discriminating variables change from study to study, those differences that have occurred between hyperactives and normal controls favor the underarousal hypothesis. In fact, only the Laufer et al. (1957) data support the overarousal proposal. In addition, it is noteworthy that the most consistent finding is that differences have usually emerged while subjects performed some cognitive task. This suggests that there are more profitable avenues for research than a continued search for a deficit in generalized CNS arousal. In fact, over a decade ago, Lacey (1967) made some strong statements regarding unitary concepts of arousal that are germane in this context. He indicated that ". . . electrocortical arousal, autonomic arousal, and behavioral arousal may be considered to be different forms of arousal, each complex in itself," thus, ". . . one cannot easily use one form of arousal as a highly valid index of another." He argued that somatic-somatic and somatic-behavioral dissociations that mitigate against a unitary concept of arousal can occur. Furthermore, he proposed that ". . . activation processes do not reflect just the intensive dimension of behavior but also the intended aim or goal of the behavior." He concluded that there is strong neurophysiological evidence that ". . . different fractions of autonomic, electroencephalographic, and motor response are mediated separately by perhaps 'intimately related' but clearly dissociable mechanisms." Lacey's admonitions have a pointed relevance to our endeavor.

Two recent proposals appear to possess more potential for understanding hyperactivity than the generalized arousal hypotheses. In a review of studies carried out in his laboratory, Conners (1976) argued persuasively that it is possible to dissociate arousal and attention in assessing the effect of stimulant drugs. He interpreted the accumulated data as indicating that stimulants act to improve selective attention rather than directly altering arousal levels. These drugs then will be useful in treating children (including hyperactive children) whose learning deficiencies are due to impairments of selective attention (central inhibition). Conners suggested that any effects of the drugs on general arousal level are secondary to their main effect on attention. The findings of Sroufe et al. (1973) and Porges et al. (1975) support this type of analysis. It is noteworthy that the evoked potential investigations reporting stimulant effects (Prichep et al., 1976; Halliday et al., 1976) implicated components of the evoked response that have been linked with attention and selective attention (Picton and Low, 1971; Picton and Hillyard, 1974; Schwent and Hillyard, 1975; Picton et al., 1978). Furthermore, the work of E. Roy John and his colleagues (1977) indicates that, as researchers acquire more sophistication in relating cortical evoked responses to cognitive processes, we may possess new and more powerful tools to define both the deficits of hyperactive children and the mechanisms responsible for the ameliorative action of stimulant drugs.

From an integration of animal and human literatures, Porges (1976) explains hyperactivity as a disorder of the balance of the antagonistic components of the autonomic nervous system—the catecholaminergically mediated sympathetic system versus the cholinergically mediated parasympathetic system. The hyperactive child represents a balance reflecting sympathetic dominance. This sympathetic dominance interferes with a proposed parasympathetic response necessary for sustained attention and thus produces hyperactive behavior. Stimulant drugs (catecholamine agonists) have their effect by eliciting a cholinergic rebound that may facilitate mediated inhibitory behaviors. Porges developed a measure of autonomic balance, and provided data showing that hyperactive children have dominant sympathetic systems relative to normal controls. Furthermore, his results show that methylphenidate selectively influences autonomic balance in the direction of normal subjects and that the dosages most effective behaviorally have the greatest "normalizing" influence on the autonomic nervous system. Although these findings need to be replicated, the model is intriguing in its link with other psychopathologies and in the possibilities it offers for understanding the mechanisms mediating hyperactivity and other attention-related problems. Initially, it also appears to provide a method for individually determining the type and dosage of pharmacological intervention that will be most effective for a given child.

NEUROCHEMICAL MODELS

Because of a possible hereditary component in hyperactivity (Wender, 1978), the respectable efficacy of pharmacological treatments for this syndrome (Oettinger, 1977), and the heuristic rewards reaped from neurochemical models of other behavioral abnormalities such as schizophrenia (Carlsson, 1978; Kornetsky and Markowitz, 1978), the temptation to speculate on similar types of models for hyperactivity is irresistable. Such speculation has yet to reach fruition, however; of the two main neurochemical hypotheses (a serotonin deficit or a cate-cholaminergic dysfunction), only one model, which postulates dysfunction of the putative brain neurotransmitter dopamine (Shaywitz, Yager, and Klopper, 1976; Shaywitz, Cohen, and Shaywitz, 1978), has some support.

The Serotonin Hypothesis

On the basis of reports of serotonin (5-hydroxytryptamine) dysfunction in other psychiatric syndromes and the diverse facilitating effects of amphetamine on monoamine function, Coleman (1971) speculated that low brain serotonin may cause hyperactivity. In support of this she reported that total blood hydroxyindoles in a heterogeneous sample of hyperactive children were below the normal level established from an unspecified group of outpatients. Subsequently, Greenberg and Coleman (1976) reported low blood 5-hydroxyindole levels in hyperactive, institutionalized mentally retarded patients. The comparison norm was established from age- and sex-matched noninstitutionalized volunteers. Furthermore, they attempted to show that medications that alleviated the hyperactive behavior tended to normalize 5-hydroxyindole levels.

There are obvious criticisms of this research, such as the uncontrolled effects of diet and institutionalization. The great majority of blood hydroxyindoles arise from the gut—how is this parameter related to brain serotonin function? Furthermore, the children in this experiment were clearly different from those now classified as suffering from hyperactivity (or MBD) and hence the data may be of little relevance.

More crucially, however, this serotonin dysfunction hypothesis, except for a report by Kløve and Bu (unpublished data) of low blood serotonin in a "true" hyperactive sample and Wender's finding of low levels (1969), has not been supported by other laboratories. Rapoport et al. (1975) found normal platelet serotonin concentrations, and normal levels of the serotonin metabolite 5-hydroxyindoleacetic acid have been reported in the urine of a MBD sample (Wender et al., 1971).

The best measures of the neurochemical status of the intact human brain are derived from assays of cerebrospinal fluid, particularly those conducted after the subject has been pretreated with the drug probenecid. Probenecid slows the efflux of certain monoamine metabolites from the cerebrospinal fluid. Serotonin metabolite levels in the cerbrospinal fluid of hyperactive children have been reported to be no different from control levels when the assay is done in conjunction with probenecid pretreatment (Shaywitz, Cohen, and Bowers, 1977) and without it (Shetty and Chase, 1976).

It seems that the relationship between hyperactivity and serotonin is not secure, although a correlation exists between total blood hydroxyindoles and hyperactivity. If we assume that it cannot be explained by confounding factors such as diet, institutionalization, medication, differential stress responses, etc., then we might expect aspects of plasma tryptophan levels to also be related to MBD. Several recent findings also suggested this hypothesis. First, brain levels of serotonin are determined by dietary intake of the serotonin precursor tryptophan (Fernstrom and Wurtman, 1971; Wurtman and Fernstrom, 1975). Second, Feingold (1973) has suggested that hyperactivity can be ameliorated by elimination of certain food additives, some of which are the salicylates. Salicylates can affect brain serotonin levels by reducing the binding of tryptophan to certain blood proteins. This effect on the brain seems to occur because tryptophan must be bound to protein carriers in order for it to pass the blood-brain barrier. Free (unbound) tryptophan does not gain access. Thus, the ratio of free to bound plasma tryptophan is inversely related to the availability of tryptophan for the brain (Tagliomonte et al., 1973).

An alternative formulation is that brain tryptophan (and hence serotonin) level is directly related to the ratio of total (free plus bound) plasma tryptophan to free tryptophan. To test the hypothesis that this ratio may be different in hyperactives, we recently compared free and total plasma tryptophan (and plasma cortisol) in 49 hyperactive children, 15 learning-disabled children (not hyperactive), and 11 children diagnosed as normal (Ferguson, Peters, Pappas, and Trites, unpublished data). There were no between-group differences on any variable. Since there were sex differences, the 17 female subjects were removed and the analyses redone—again no differences were observed. A selected group of hyperactives scoring "high" on the Conners scales (parents and teachers) were compared with age-matched hyperactives scoring low, with another group diagnosed as having learning disability, and with normals—again there were no significant effects. In addition, all possible correlations were run for the three groups together on the three blood analysis variables plus the age, hyperactivity, and conduct problem factors of the mother's and teacher's Conners questionnaires. From all of these analyses there were no significant effects. Subsequently we compared 13 selected hyperactive boys with 13 age-matched learning-disabled boys on free and total plasma tryptophan, blood serotonin, plasma protein, and plasma cortisol. There were no significant differences even when the groups were reduced to the seven most severe hyperactives and their age matches. Finally, we compared samples from eight hyperactive boys on Ritalin versus placebo. Samples were collected and assays done under double-blind conditions. The same five variables were analyzed once again, with no significant differences emerging. There is no ready explanation for the conflict between the data of Coleman (1971) and Kløve and Bu (unpublished) and our data. The lack of significant findings is discouraging for the Coleman serotonin hypothesis and has led us to abandon these blood analyses as a way of subgrouping hyperactive children.

Catecholamine Hypotheses

The proliferation of anatomical, developmental, and behavioral surveys on the catecholamines made it inevitable that someone postulate a catecholaminergic basis. There are two forms of the catecholamine hypothesis. The first (Wender, 1974) attributed MBD to functional underactivity of norepinephrine systems, and the second (Shaywitz, Yager, and Klopper, 1976) attributed it to dopamine deficiency.

Linking research on the role of the catecholamines in rodent behavior to MBD, Wender cautiously suggested that a genetically determined underactivity of noradrenergic reward-arousal systems determines MBD. Amphetamine and other stimulants are effective symptomatic treatments, he speculated, because they enhance activity in these systems. The hypothesis has not been supported—it is not clear that noradrenalin is the transmitter exclusively involved in reward (Stein, 1978) or arousal (Robinson, Vanderwolf, and Pappas, 1977) processes in the rodent. In addition, the levels of urinary norepinephrine and its metabolites have not been found to differ between children with MBD and a control group (Wender et al., 1971), although this negative finding is scarcely crucial for the norephinephrine hypothesis.

The ideal experiment would examine norepinephrine metabolite levels in the cerebrospinal fluid of children pretreated with probenecid, which retards metabolite outflow. However, this procedure does entail discomfort and risk. Alternatively, it has been suggested that urinary levels of the metabolite 3-methoxy-4-hydroxymandelic acid (MHPG) fairly accurately reflect brain norepinephrine activity (Maas and Landis, 1971). However, Wender et al. (1971) reported no correlation of MBD with the level of this metabolite in urine.

One potentially valuable observation here is that, in a group of hyperactive children, the extent of minor physical anomalies (stigmata) correlated significantly with ratings of hyperactivity and conduct problems (Rapoport, Quinn, and Lamprecht, 1974), although the correlations were not large (0.28 and 0.35, respectively). Stigmata scores were also positively correlated ($r = 0.38$) with plasma levels of dopamine β-hydroxylase, the enzyme that converts dopamine to norepinephrine. The majority of this enzyme in plasma probably derives from peripheral autonomic nerve endings, although it is not unreasonable to suggest that this level may also index its activity in the brain.

Quinn and Rapoport (1974) also uncovered a positive correlation between stigmata and retrospective reports of paternal hyperactivity. More recently, Waldrop et al. (1978) reported that the presence of minor physical anomalies in boys at birth signficantly correlated with objective ratings of MBD symptoms at 3 years of age. These data are consistent with the notion of some genetic determination and bolster the suspicion for some neurochemical translation of this determination.

Although there is no evidence to support either a serotonergic or noradrenergic mechanism for MBD, Shaywitz, Yager, and Klopper (1976) and Shaywitz et al. (1976, 1978) have put forward a dopamine dysfunction hypothesis. Their supporting evidence from metabolite studies on children is not compelling, but a rat analog has also been offered.

The major metabolite of dopamine is homovanillic acid (HVA). In the three experiments that have compared resting HVA levels between control subjects and MBD children, no differences have been found. These experiments have examined levels in urine (Wender et al., 1971), cerebrospinal fluid (Shetty and Chase, 1976) and cerebrospinal fluid after probenecid pretreatment (Shaywitz et al., 1977). Shetty and Chase reported that d-amphetamine improved the behavior of 10 children and also lowered their HVA levels—the correlation between improvement and reduction in HVA level was very high ($r = 0.91, p < 0.001$). On the basis of this, they felt that their data supported the hypothesis of dopamine pathology in MBD. Close examination of their data, however, shows that baseline HVA levels in the 10 hyperactives who received amphetamine were 190% of those in children who received placebo. This difference barely fails to reach significance ($t = 2.01, 0.05 < p < 0.10$) by our calculations. After from 2 to 14 days of treatment, HVA levels in the placebo group did not differ from baseline, while those in the amphetamine group significantly declined by 34% to a level equal to that of the placebo group. It seems that the factor that produced an effect here was the inflated predrug score of the d-amphetamine group, which occurred despite random assignment. Whatever the reason for this unusually high level, it would naturally be expected to decline.

This would produce the observed correlation between degree of HVA decline and behavioral improvement, since d-amphetamine causes the latter.

In the experiment by Shaywitz et al. (1977), cerebrospinal fluid HVA levels were not found to differ between 26 controls and six MBD children. Levels of HVA (and 5-hydroxyindoleacetic acid) were, however, significantly correlated with probenecid levels. Since probenecid levels were 47% higher in the MBD sample, a correction for this was employed. The ratio of HVA to probenecid was calculated for each subject. This ratio was found to be significantly lower for the MBD sample. However, it is equivocal as to whether this ratio reflects the HVA or the probenecid factor. One could justifiably argue for a defect in probenecid clearance in the MBD sample.

The safest conclusion from the research examined is that there is no compelling evidence for any form of monoamine hypothesis for MBD. More measurements of monoamines and their metabolites, particularly in cerebrospinal fluid, are required, along with less data twisting to provide significant effects. This data collection is arduous for both experimenter and subject. New, more sensitive methods of assay that also permit a greater number of substances to be assayed in a single sample may provide the key. Beyond this, however, one is also faced with the difficult problem of disentangling correlations to discern causations. Two final caveats are warranted. Dopaminergic systems are sensitive to transient perturbations, perhaps especially so for the developing brain (Lundborg, 1972; Ahlenius et al., 1977). It must be demonstrated that lingering effects that result from the actions of stimulants on dopamine function cannot account for the differences observed between MBD and control samples. Second, although the evidence is best for some alteration of dopamine systems in hyperactivity, dopamine hypotheses are ubiquitous. Forms have been invoked to account for schizophrenia (Carlsson, 1978) as well as extrapyramidal syndromes (Barbeau, 1978). The supporting evidence for these is considerably more compelling than that offered for hyperactivity. As familiarity has been argued to breed contempt, so may ubiquity breed the suspicion that some general, but not essential, factor may be operating to produce the correlations.

ANIMAL MODELS

Increased motor activity has been shown to occur after chronic lead ingestion in developing rats (Silbergeld and Goldberg, 1974, 1976; Sobotka and Cook, 1974; Kostas, McFarland, and Drew, 1976;

Overmann, 1977). It has also been reported that d-amphetamine reduces this hyperactivity (Kostas et al., 1976). In support of this model, hair samples of children diagnosed as learning disabled reportedly show elevated lead and cadmium content (Pihl and Parkes, 1977). Extensive discussions of this lead model and some of its methodological problems have recently been presented elsewhere (Goldberg and Silbergeld, 1977; Michaelson et al., 1977; Breese et al., 1978).

Two recent alternative approaches that also show promise are those of Campbell and Randall (1975, 1977) and Shaywitz, Yager, and Klopper (1976). The Campbell and Randall model is based on a normal, maturation-linked hyperactivity that is elicited in the young rat by separation from other rats. The model of Shaywitz, Yager, and Klopper (1976) is based on behavioral disturbances in the young rat after a permanent but moderate depletion of brain dopamine by injection of the neurotoxin 6-hydroxydopamine.

The Ontogenetic Model

Rats display a short-lived period of locomotor hyperactivity around 15 days of age (Campbell, Lytle, and Fibiger, 1969). This hyperactivity is elicited by isolation of the pup in an unfamiliar environment (Campbell and Raskin, 1978; Dollinger and Raskin, 1978). It was originally suggested by Campbell et al. (1969) that this hyperactivity reflected an earlier ontogeny for excitatory, brainstem catecholaminergic circuits than for inhibitory, forebrain cholinergic circuits. Recent data have led Campbell and Raskin (1978) to abandon this simple sequential caudal-to-rostral development of excitatory and inhibitory centers in the rat brain. However, there is research support for the notion of late (15–25 days postnatal) maturation of the cholinergic circuits (Fibiger, Lytle, and Campbell, 1970; Moorcroft, 1971). Another earlier-developing inhibitory process, mediated by serotonin, may also mature at about 15 days (Mabry and Campbell, 1974).

Contrary to what would be predicted from this schema, chemically induced lesions of norepinephrine (Pappas et al., 1975) or dopamine (Shaywitz, Yager, and Klopper, 1976; Shaywitz et al., 1976) neurons in the developing rat do not attenuate this hyperactivity (in fact the latter exacerbates it). Nevertheless, an attractive rat model for human hyperactivity would be offered if this phenomenon accurately paralleled processes in MBD.

Neither d-amphetamine (Campbell et al., 1969; Sobrian, Weltman, and Pappas, 1975) nor methylphenidate (Pappas, Gallivan, Dugas, and Saari, in preparation) "calms" the hyperkinetic 15-day-old rat. In fact, both drugs increase activity levels. However, if the rat is confined to an apparatus that contains an anesthetized adult rat, then d-amphetamine has an entirely different behavioral effect—the rat's locomotion is not increased (Campbell and Randall, 1975, 1977). Rather, it spends its time in contact with the anesthetized adult, and, if the latter is mechanically moved, pursues the adult. This behavior at 15 days contrasts with that at 30, when the amphetamine response is not determined by the presence of the adult—the drug produces activity under isolation or in the presence of the adult, although the drug is not nearly as effective as at 15 days. In the 30-day-old rat, d-amphetamine reduces contact time with the adult.

These observations led Campbell and Randall to postulate the following processes in rat and human. Reflexive, nonspecific, biologically significant behaviors are the first to mature. These are organized at the brainstem and limbic system level. With maturation, forebrain areas such as the cortex and hippocampus begin to modulate these behaviors. To explain the differential amphetamine response in 15- and 30-day-old rats, Campbell and Randall suggest that the drug activates these biologically relevant behaviors in the younger rat. That is, it arouses behavior and canalizes it toward other rats if these are in the environment. With brain maturation, the drug simply produced heightened excitation that is not specifically directed. Finally, they suggest that hyperactivity may represent a developmental lag in the transition from infantile to adult response to amphetamine, which would explain the "paradoxical" effects of d-amphetamine, such as directed attention toward adults.

This is a provocative model. The effects of amphetamine in hyperactivity, however, are not paradoxical, but probably reflect the same process that the drug produces in normal children. Normal prepubertal boys respond to d-amphetamine as do hyperactive boys—with improved performance on cognitive tasks and with reduced motor activity (Rapoport et al., 1978). In the terms of the Campbell-Randall model, this implies that what may distinguish the hyperactive child from his normal age peer is his relative inability to canalize his behavior in the absence of stimulant drugs. Thus, one wonders what brain manipulations would induce hyperactivity in the young rat both in the absence and especially in the presence of other rats. Would stimulants reduce hyperactivity in the latter case?

In addition, it is questionable whether, with maturation, the dysfunctions of MBD tend to abate (Wender, 1978). Wood et al. (1976) identified a group of adults with MBD-like symptoms. As compared with placebo in a double-blind study, methylphenidate significantly improved self-ratings on scales measuring anxiety, energy level, attention, and temperament. This could require another revision to the model—although children with MBD may indeed suffer from a maturational lag, they also may never catch up.

The Dopamine Dysfunction Model

Shaywitz, Yager, and Klopper (1976) have reported that chronic lowering of dopamine levels in the neonatal rat by intracisternal injection of the neurotoxin 6-hydroxydopamine exaggerates the hyperactivity observed around 15–25 days of age. On the basis of these and other data, it was suggested that this dopamine dysfunction syndrome in the rat could serve as an analog for MBD. Shaywitz et al. (1977) had attempted to support this concept with studies of cerebrospinal fluid metabolites in children; however, the results of this and other research were equivocal. A successful rat model would considerably reinforce this dopamine hypothesis. Shaywitz et al. injected their rats at 5 days of age; these animals were more hyperactive than controls between 15 and 22 days of age. Although this effect abated, the rats showed a severe deficit in an active avoidance task when tested at 27 days of age. This pattern of behavioral effects was argued to be analogous to the maturational disappearance of hyperactivity in maturing MBD children with the persistence of various cognitive, perceptual, and emotional difficulties.

This rat model has been criticized on methodological and interpretive grounds by several research groups (Kalat, 1976; McLean, Kostrzewa, and May, 1976; Pappas, Ferguson, and Saari, 1976). In addition to these published critiques, it is important to note that, although the hyperactivity after dopamine depletion is a replicable finding (Pappas, Gallivan, Dugas, and Saari, in preparation), juvenile hyperactivity is also caused by neonatal brain 5-hydroxytryptamine depletion (Breese, Vogel, and Mueller, 1978), and to a lesser extent by norepinephrine depletion (Pappas et al., 1975).

Subsequent to their demonstration of hyperactivity in dopamine-depleted infant rats, Shaywitz et al. (1976) reported that d-amphetamine significantly reduced activity levels at 22 and 26 days of age. This effect, they argued, paralleled the so-called paradoxical response to this drug in children with MBD. As pointed out earlier, Rapoport et al. (1978) have quashed the notion that stimulants have a paradoxical effect in MBD. Rather, the effects of stimulants in normal children seem similar to those in hyperactive children. Yet, the stimulants markedly exacerbate the existing hyperactivity in normal developing rats (Campbell et al., 1969; Sobrian et al., 1975) and in the study of Shaywitz et al. (1976) significantly elevated activity at several ages in the control rats. This diversity between human and rat effects is not crucial to the Shaywitz model. Potentially more troublesome, however, is that in our laboratory both *d*-amphetamine and methylphenidate substantially elevated activity in young dopamine-depleted rats (Pappas, Gallivan, Dugas, and Saari, in preparation). Differing techniques may explain this discrepancy. For example, in our laboratory the 6-hydroxydopamine injections are administered through the lateral ventricles on days 1 and 2 of life. The rats in the Yale laboratories were injected on day 5 through the cisterna magna. The extent and pattern of dopamine depletions may differ from these two techniques.

Despite this difference in the activity responses to stimulants, other aspects of our data agree with the dopamine depletion model. As Shaywitz, Yager, and Klopper (1976) had reported for avoidance learning at 27 days of age, so were our dopamine-depleted rats markedly inferior to controls on a two-way shuttle avoidance task during adulthood. The administration of *d*-amphetamine (2 mg/kg), however, significantly improved avoidance learning in these rats to a level equivalent to that of saline-injected controls. This improvement would be predicted from the dopamine depletion model.

Further research is required to resolve the discrepancies between laboratories for stimulant effects in the young dopamine-depleted animal. In this regard it is important to note that the hyperactivity displayed by young rats after neonatal 5-hydroxytryptamine depletion is not corrected but exacerbated by *d*-amphetamine (G. R. Breese, personal communication).

Animal Models: Concluding Comments

Insults to the developing organism, whether toxicological (e.g., lead), pharmacological (e.g., 6-hydroxydopamine), or otherwise (anoxia, x-ray irradiation), may have their greatest altering effect on neural systems that are in the process of development or that subsequently develop. Thus, late postnatal–maturing brain structures such as the hippocampus and cerebellum may be more affected than structures where development occurs mainly in the later gestational periods. Hence, although diverse insults may yield some diverse behavioral consequences because of specificities of neural effects, they may also produce some common effects because they act on vulnerable substrates. Thus, a variety of early treatments could commonly alter susceptible systems by arresting growth, suppressing appetite, affecting maternal-infant interactions, etc. One general result may be juvenile hyperactivity.

This does not negate those manipulations as models of MBD. Indeed, hyperactivity may be a prepotent behavioral outcome of many types of perturbations of the developing brain. This would agree with the multiplicity of etiologies for childhood hyperactivity.

There are also alternative approaches. Perhaps the focus for animal models has been aimed too often at the supposed kinetic component of MBD. The hypermotile infant rat may in fact poorly approximate the hyperactive child because hypermotility is not a clearly established aspect of the syndrome (Werry and Sprague, 1970; Douglas, 1972). Changing the focus requires a shift in assumptions about what criteria must be met by a model of MBD. The most explicit exposition of criteria has been outlined by Shaywitz (1976):

1. The animal model must mimic central features of MBD
2. The animal and human syndromes must have similar pathogeneses
3. The animal syndrome must be evident during early development
4. Stimulants (and other drugs found effective in MBD) must ameliorate the animal syndrome

The first criterion is the most obvious, but perhaps the most difficult to correctly satisfy, since it requires assumptions about what salient behaviors are to be modeled. As pointed out earlier, the most frequently selected feature has been hyperkinesis, but this is not in fact a readily verifiable element of MBD. The second criterion seems less of a criterion than an aim of the modeling process. The third criterion is desirable but unnecessary. Models that successfully mimic other syndromes have not necessarily adhered to requirements about maturational status. For example, Parkinson's disease manifests itself with advancing age, yet the most successful animal model derives from observations of the effects of disruption of certain dopamine pathways in the rat brain. This rat model, in which age is not a variable, reproduces many of the neurochemical abnormalities observed in Parkinsonian patients and can also be used to predict pharmacotherapies that ultimately prove beneficial in the disease (Ungerstedt, 1974). The fourth criterion ought to be the most important. Thus, a potentially applicable model for MBD would be one in which an animal behavioral abnormality that resembles a presumptive component of MBD is attenuated by stimulant drugs. Then, inferences about the mechanisms of action of the drug and of the behavioral abnormality can be compared with data from children with MBD. Two recent models are elaborated below, principally because of their satisfaction of the fourth criterion. In both models, behaviors other than hyperactivity were the focal symptoms.

As part of a fascinating series of neo-Pavlovian experiments that have yielded various canine behavioral syndromes, eight dogs who were untrainable were identified (Arnold et al., 1973; Corson et al., 1973; Corson et al., 1976). These dogs reacted with extreme agitation to attempted restraint in a Pavlovian stand. This behavior did not extinguish and, as a result, these animals could not undergo conditioning procedures. The administration of d-amphetamine (in clinically relevant doses of 0.2–1.0 mg/kg) had a marked calming effect on these "hyperkinetic" dogs. This effect was sufficient to permit the dogs to undergo the Pavlovian training and to successfully learn conditional leg flexion responses. These investigators suggested that these dogs were analogous to hyperkinetic children and that the term hyperkinetic syndrome actually should be replaced by hypoinhibitory syndrome (Corson et al., 1976), which they suggested was more descriptive of the abnormality. They felt that the condition resulted from a deficit in catecholaminergic activity in inhibitory brain circuits, which amphetamines supposedly corrected.

This research is presented in a semi-anecdotal fashion and certainly merits follow-up. In particular, more adequate behavioral measures are required to determine the extent of the similarity between these dogs and children with MBD. Incidentally, these investigators reported that the d-isomer of amphetamine was more potent than the l-isomer. Based on data that suggested that the d-isomer was more effective for norepinephrine-releasing brain systems whereas the isomers were equieffective for norepinephrine and dopamine systems (e.g., Taylor and Snyder, 1970), these investigators suggested that the relevant catecholamine was norepinephrine. More recent data disagree with this distinction between the isomers (Bunney et al., 1975) and invalidate this suggestion.

Another more recent model has attempted to mimic in the rat the poor impulse control displayed by hyperactive children (Pappas et al., 1978). In this experiment, water-deprived rats were trained to drink water in an apparatus and then exposed to brief electric shocks delivered through the spout, contingent on licking. Normal rats learned to inhibit drinking after about seven to eight shocks. Prior injection of the minor tranquilizer chlordiazepoxide (Librium, 8 mg/kg) more than doubled the number of shocks that the rats were willing to receive. The supposition here was that this disinhibition of punished behavior mimics the attenuated impulse control in MBD. (Relevant to this supposition is the fact that minor tranquilizers do not reduce the symptoms of hyperactive children.) In the experiment, the stimulants d-amphetamine and methylphenidate counteracted this chlordiazepoxide-induced disinhibition in a dose-related manner. They also tended to reduce the number of shocks received in control rats who were not pretreated with chlordiazepoxide. Figure 1 shows the effects of *d*-amphetamine. Future research should further assess the possibility that antagonism of this disinhibition by drugs reflect their clinical efficacy for symptomatic treatment of

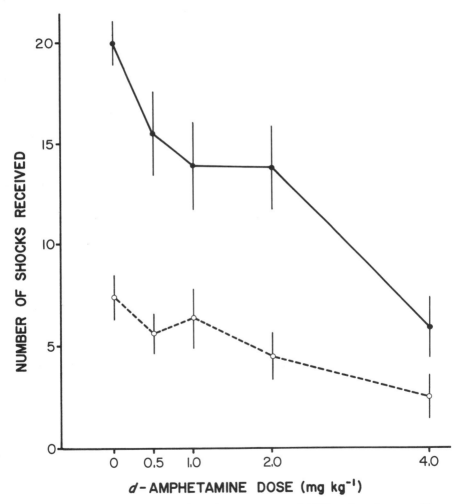

Figure 1.   The effects of *d*-amphetamine on response inhibition in saline- or chlor-diazepoxide-pretreated rats. The ordinate shows the mean number of shocks received by the various groups in a punishment paradigm. Chlordiazepoxide-treated rats, ——; saline-treated rats, – – –. As the figure shows, chlordiazepoxide greatly increased the number of shocks received. This effect was counteracted in a dose-related fashion by *d*-amphetamine.

hyperactivity. In this respect, it is worth noting that phenobarbital, which is contraindicated for hyperactivity (Eisenberg, 1966), synergized with chlordiazepoxide in this test of impulse control and also by itself significantly attenuated impulse control. Second, the developing rat does not perform well in passive avoidance tasks (Riccio, Rohrbaugh, and Hodges, 1968; Blosovski, Cudennec, and Garrigou, 1977) These tasks are also sensitive to the rat's capacity for impulse control. If the young rat's performance on such tasks is improved by stimulants, this would not only support the model but also add a developmental component.

We conclude that whether or not a successful animal model can be found for a syndrome as complex as childhood hyperactivity is yet to be determined. These endeavors will, however, ultimately increase our understanding of brain-behavior relationships. Furthermore, the unraveling of the ontogeny of neurochemical systems has only recently begun. In many systems, although maturation varies monotonically with age, there are distinct inflection points (e.g., Coyle and Enna, 1976; Pardo et al., 1977). In other systems there may be points of transition at which development occurs suddenly (e.g., Compochiaro and Coyle, 1978). Identifying a correlation between this and behavioral maturation, such as can be demonstrated for some anatomically specified elements and behavior (Goldman, 1976), is a clear possibility. The relevance of this to the types of conjecture about the basis of hyperactivity that we have encountered is obvious.

REFERENCES

Ahlenius, S., Engel, J., Hard, E., Larsson, K., Lunborg, P., and Sinnerstedt, P. 1977. Open field behavior and gross motor development in offspring of nursing rat mothers given penfluridol. Pharmacol. Biochem. Behav. 6:343–347.

Arnold, L. E., Kirilcuk, V., Corson, S. A., and Corson, E. O. 1973. Levoamphetamine and dextroamphetamine: Differential effect on aggression and hyperkinesis in children and dogs. Am. J. Psychiatry 130:165–170.

Barbeau, A. 1978. The last ten years of progress in the clinical pharmacology of the extrapyramidal system. In M. A. Lipton, A. Dimascio, and K. F. Killam (eds.), Psychopharmacology: A Generation of Progress, pp. 771–776. Raven Press, New York.

Barkley, R. A., and Jackson, T. L. 1977. Hyperkinesis, autonomic nervous system activity, stimulant drug effects. J. Child Psychol. Psychiatry 18:347–357.

Blosovski, D., Cudennec, A., and Garrigon, D. 1977. Deficits in passive avoidance learning following atropine in the developing rat. Psychopharmacology 54:139–143.

Boydstun, J. A., Ackerman, P. T., Stevens, D. A., Clements, S. D., Peters, J. F., and Dykman, R. A. 1968. Physiologic and motor conditioning and generalization in children with minimal brain dysfunction. Conditional Reflex 3:81–104.

Bradley, C. 1937. The behavior of children receiving benzedrine. Am. J. Psychiatry 44:577–585.

Breese, G. R., Mueller, R. A., Mailman, R. B., Frye, G. D. and Vogel, R. A. 1978. Study of drug mechanisms and disease symptoms in animals: An alternative to animal models of CNS disorders. Neuropsychopharmacology. In press.

Breese, G. R., Vogel, R. A., and Mueller, R. A. 1978. Biochemical and behavioral alterations in developing rats treated with 5,7-dihydroxytryptamine. J. Pharmacol. Exp. Ther. 205:587–595.

Buchsbaum, M., and Wender, P. H. 1973. Average evoked responses in normal and minimally brain dysfunctioned children treated with amphetamine. Arch. Gen. Psychiatry 29:764–770.

Buckley, R. E. 1972. A neurophysiological proposal for the amphetamine response in hyperkinetic children. Psychosomatics 13:93–99.

Bunney, B. S., Walters, J. R., Kuhar, M. J., Roth, R. H., and Aghajanian, G. K. 1975. D and L Amphetamine stereoisomers: Comparative potencies in affecting the firing of central dopaminergic and noradrenergic neurons. Psychopharmacol. Commun. 1:177–190.

Campbell, B. A., Lytle, L. D., and Fibiger, H. C. 1969. Ontogeny of arousal and cholinergic inhibitory mechanisms in the rat. Science 166:637–638.

Campbell, B. A., and Randall, P. K. 1975. Paradoxical effects of amphetamine on behavioral arousal in neonatal and adult rats: A possible animal model of the calming effect of amphetamine on hyperkinetic children. In N. R. Ellis (ed.), Aberrant Development in Infancy, pp. 104–112. Lawrence Erlbaum Associates, Hillsdale, New Jersey.

Campbell, B. A., and Randall, P. J. 1977. Paradoxical effects of amphetamine on preweaning and postweaning rats. Science 195:888–891.

Campbell, B. A., and Raskin, L. A. 1978. Ontogeny of behavioral arousal: The role of environmental stimuli. J. Comp. Physiol. Psychol. 92:176–184.

Capute, A., Niedermeyer, E., and Richardson, F. 1968. The electroencephalogram in children with minimal cerebral dysfunction. Pediatrics 41:1104–1114.

Carlsson, A. 1978. Antipsychotic drugs, neurotransmitters and schizophrenia. Am. J. Psychiatry 135:164–173.

Clements, S. D., and Peters, J. E. 1962. Minimal brain dysfunctions in the school age child. Arch. Gen. Psychiatry 6:185–197.

Cohen, N. J., and Douglas, V. I. 1972. Characteristics of the orienting response in hyperactive and normal children. Psychophysiology 9:238–245.

Cohen, N. J., Douglas, V. I., and Morgenstern, G. 1971. The effect of methylphenidate on attentive behavior and autonomic activity in hyperactive children. Psychopharmacologia 22:282–294.

Coleman, M. 1971. Serotonin concentration in whole blood of hyperactive children. J. Pediatr. 78:985.

Coleman, M. 1973. Serotonin and central nervous system syndromes of childhood. A review. J. Autism Child. Schizophr. 3:27–35.

Compochiaro, P., and Coyle, J. T. 1978. Ontogenetic development of Kainate neurotoxicity: correlates with glutamatergic innervation. Proc. Natl. Acad. Sci. U.S.A. 75:2025–2029.

Conners, C. K. 1972. Stimulant drugs and cortical evoked responses in learning and behavior disorders in children. In W. L. Smith (ed.), Drugs, Development and Cerebral Function, p. 179. Charles C Thomas, Springfield, Ill.

Conners, C. K. 1976. Learning disabilities and stimulant drugs in children: Theoretical implications. In R. M. Knights and D. J. Bakker (eds.), The Neuropsychology of Learning Disorders, pp. 389–404. University Park Press, Baltimore.

Conners, C. K., and Rothschild, G. H. 1973. The effect of dextroamphetamine on habituation of peripheral vascular response in children. J. Abnorm. Child Psychol. 1:16–25.

Corson, S. A., Corson, E. O'L., Kirilcuk, V., Kirilcuk, J., Knopp, W., and Arnold, L. E. 1973. Differential effects of amphetamines on clinically relevant dog models of hyperkinesis and stereotypic relevance to Huntington's chorea. Adv. Neurol. 1:681–697.

Corson, S. A., Corson, E. O'L., Arnold, L. E., and Knopp, W. 1976. Animal models of violence and hyperkinesis: Interaction of psychopharmacologic and psychosocial therapy in behavior modification. In G. Serban and A. Kling (eds.), Animal Models in Human Psychobiology, pp. 111–139. Plenum Press, New York.

Coyle, J. T., and Enna, S. J. 1976. Neurochemical aspects of the ontogenesis of gabanergic neurons in the rat brain. Brain Res. 3:119–133.

Dollinger, M. J., and Raskin, L. A. 1978. Effect of olfactory bulbectomy on reactivity to environmental stimuli in the preweaning rat. Paper presented at the Annual Meeting of the Eastern Psychological Association, Washington, D.C.

Douglas, V. I. 1972. Stop, Look and Listen: The problem of sustained attention and impulse control in hyperactive and normal children. Can. J. Behav. Sci. 4:259–282.

Duffy, E. 1962. Activation and Behavior. John Wiley & Sons, Inc., New York.

Dykman, R. A., Ackerman, P. T., Clements, S. D., and Peters, J. E. 1971. Specific learning disabilities: An attentional deficit syndrome. In H. R. Myklebust (ed.), Progress in Learning Disabilities, Vol. 2, pp. 56–93. Grune and Stratton, New York.

Eisenberg, L. 1966. The management of the hyperkinetic child. Dev. Med. Child Neurol. 8:593–598.

Feingold, B. B. 1973. Introduction to Clinical Allergy. Charles C Thomas, Springfield, Ill.

Ferguson, H., Simpson, S., and Trites, R. 1976. Psychophysiological study of methylphenidate responders and nonresponders. In R. Knights and D. J. Bakker (eds.), Neuropsychology of Learning Disorders, pp. 89–98. University Park Press, Baltimore.

Fernstrom, J. D., and Wurtman, R. J. 1971. Brain serotonin content: Physiological dependence on plasma tryptophan levels. Science 173:149–152.

Fibiger, H. D., Lytle, L. D., and Campbell, B. A. 1970. Cholinergic modulation of adrenergic arousal in the developing rat. J. Comp. Physiol. Psychol. 72:384–389.

Firestone, P., and Douglas, V. I. 1975. The effects of reward and punishment on reaction times and autonomic activity in hyperactive and normal children. J. Abnorm. Child Psychol. 3:201–216.

Freibergs, V., and Douglas, V. I. 1969. Concept learning in hyperactive and normal children. J. Abnorm. Psychol. 74:388–395.

Goldberg, A. M., and Silbergeld, E. K. 1977. Animal models of hyperactivity. In

I. Hanin and E. Usden (eds.), Animal Models in Psychiatry and Neurology, pp. 371–384. Pergamon Press, Inc., New York.

Goldman, P. S. 1976. Maturation of the mammalian nervous system and the ontogeny of behavior. In J. S. Rosenblatt et al. (eds.), Advances in the Study of Behavior, Vol. 7, pp. 1–90. Academic Press, New York.

Greenberg, A. S., and Coleman, M. 1976. Depressed 5-hydroxyindole levels associated with hyperactive and aggressive behavior: Relationship to drug response. Arch. Gen. Psychiatry 33:331–341.

Grunewald-Zuberbier, E., Grunewald, G., and Rasche, A. 1975. Hyperactive behavior and EEG arousal reactions in children. Electroencephalogr. Clin. Neurophysiol. 38:149–159.

Hall, R. A., Griffin, R. B., Moyer, D. L., Hopkins, K. H., and Rapoport, M. 1976. Evoked potential, stimulus intensity and drug treatment in hyperkinesis. Psychophysiology 13:405–418.

Halliday, R., Rosenthal, J. H., Naylor, H., and Callaway, E. 1976. Averaged evoked potential predictors of clinical improvement in hyperactive children treated with methylphenidate: An initial study and replication. Psychophysiology 13:429–440.

Hughes, J. R., and Myklebust, H. R. 1971. The EEG in a controlled study of minimal brain dysfunction. Electroencephalogr. Clin. Neurophysiol. 31:292.

John, E. R, Karmel, B. Z., Corning, W. C., Easton, P., Brown, D., Ahn, H., John, M., Harmony, T., Prichep, L., Toro, A., Gerson, I., Bartlett, F., Thatcher, R., Kaye, H., Valdes, P., and Schwartz, E. 1977. Neurometrics numerical taxonomy identifies different profiles of brain dysfunctions within groups of behaviorally similar people. Science 196:1393–1410.

Kahn, E., and Cohen, L. H. 1934. Organic driveness: A brainstem syndrome and an experience. N. Engl. J. Med. 210:748–756.

Kalat, J. W. 1976. Minimal brain dysfunction: dopamine depletion? Science 194:450–451.

Kløve, H., and Bu, B. 1976. The effect of ritalin on electrodermal responses, blood serotonin, and behavior in hyperkinetic children. Paper presented at the International Neuropsychology Society Meeting, February, Toronto.

Knights, R., and Hinton, C. C. 1969. The effects of methylphenidate on the motor skills and behavior of children with learning problems. J. Nerv. Ment. Dis. 148:643–654.

Knights, R. M., and Viets, C. A. 1975. Effects of Pemoline on hyperactive boys. Pharmacol. Biochem. Behav. 3:1107–1114.

Knobel, M., Wolman, M. A., and Mason, E. 1959. Hyperkinesis and organesis in children. Arch. Gen. Psychiatry 1:310–321.

Kornetsky, C., and Markowitz, R. 1978. Animal models of schizophrenia. In M. A. Lipton, A. Dimascio, and K. F. Killam (eds.), Psychopharmacology: A Generation of Progress, pp. 563–567. Raven Press, New York.

Kostas, J., McFarland, D. J., and Drew, W. G. 1976. Lead-induced hyperactivity. Chronic exposure during the neonatal period in the rat. Pharmacology 14:435–442.

Lacey, J. I. 1967. Somatic response patterning and stress: Some revisions of activation theory. In M. H. Appley and R. Trumbull (eds.), Psychological Stress: Issues in Research. Appleton-Century-Crofts, New York.

Laufer, M. W., Denhoff, E., and Solomons, S. 1957. Hyperkinetic impulse disorder in children's behavior problems. Psychosom. Med. 19:38–49.

Lundborg, P. 1972. Abnormal ontogeny in young rabbits after chronic administration of haloperidol to the nursing mothers. Brain Res. 44:684–687.

Maas, J. W., and Landis, D. H. 1971. The metabolism of circulatory norepinephrine by human subjects. J. Pharmacol. Exp. Ther. 177:600–612.

Mabry, P. D., and Campbell, B. A. 1974. Ontogeny of serotonergic inhibition of behavioral arousal in the rat. J. Comp. Physiol. Psychol. 86:193–201.

Malmo, R. B. 1959. Activation: a neuropsychological dimension. Psychol. Rev. 66:367–386.

McLean, J. H., Kostrzewa, R. M., and May, J. G. 1976. Minimal brain dysfunction: Dopamine depletion? Science 194:45.

Michaelson, I. A., Bornschein, R. L., Loch, R. K., and Ratales, L. S. 1977. Minimal brain dysfunction hyperkinesis, significance of nutritional status in animal models of hyperactivity. In I. Hanin and E. Usdin (eds.), Animal Models in Psychiatry and Neurology, pp. 37–49. Pergamon Press, Inc., New York.

Millichap, J. G. 1973. Drugs in management of minimal brain dysfunction. Academ. Sci. 205:321–334.

Milstein, V., and Small, J. G. 1974. Photic responses in "minimal brain dysfunction." Dis. Nerv. Syst. 35:355–357.

Montagu, J. 1975. The hyperactive child: A behavioral electrodermal and EEG investigation. Dev. Med. Child. Neurol. 17:299–305.

Moorcroft, W. H. 1971. Ontogeny of forebrain inhibition of behavioral arousal in the rat. Brain Res. 35:513–522.

Oettinger, L. 1977. Pediatric psychopharmacology: A review with special reference to Deanol. Dis. Nerv. Syst. 38:25–31.

Overmann, S. R. 1977. Behavioral effects of asymptomatic lead exposure during neonatal development in rats. Toxicol. Appl. Pharmacol. 41:459–471.

Pappas, B. A., Ferguson, H. B., and Saari, M. 1976. Minimal brain dysfunction: Dopamine depletion? Science 194:451–452.

Pappas, B. A., Peters, D. A. V., Sobrian, S. K., Blouin, A., and Drew, B. 1975. Early behavioral and catecholaminergic effects of 6-hydroxydopamine and guanethidine in the neonatal rat. Pharmacol. Biochem. Behav. 3:681–685.

Pappas, B. A., Vogel, R. A., Frye, G. D., Breese, G. R., and Mueller, R. A. 1978. Stimulant drugs enhance effects of punishment in normal and chlordiazepoxide treated rats. Paper presented at Society for Neuroscience Annual Meeting, St. Louis, Mo.

Pardo, J. V., Creese, I., Burt, D. A., and Snyder, S. H. 1977. Ontogenesis of dopamine receptor binding in the corpus striatum of the rat. Brain Res. 125:376–382.

Picton, T. W., Campbell, K. B., Baribeau-Braun, J., and Proulx, G. B. 1978. The neurophysiology of human attention. In J. Requin (ed.), Attention and Performance, Vol. 7. Lawrence Erlbaum Associates, Hillsdale, New Jersey. In press.

Picton, T. W., and Hillyard, S. A. 1974. Human auditory evoked potentials: Effects of attention. Electroencephalogr. Clin. Neurophysiol. 36:191–200.

Picton, T. W., and Low, M. D. 1971. The CNV and semantic content of stimuli in the experimental paradigm: Effects of feedback. Electroencephalogr. Clin. Neurophysiol. 31:451–456.

Pihl, R. O., and Parkes, M. 1977. Hair element content in learning disabled children. Science 198:204–206.

Porges, S. W. 1976. Peripheral and neurochemical parallels of psychopathology. A psychophysiological model relating autonomic imbalance to hyperactivity, psychopathy and autism. In H. W. Reese (ed.), Advances in Child Behavior and Development, Vol. 2. Academic Press, New York.

Porges, S. W., Walter, G. F., Korb, R. J., and Sprague, R. L. 1975. The influences of methylphenidate on heart rate and behavioral measures at attention in hyperactive children. Child Dev. 46:727–733.

Prichep, L. S., Sutton, S., and Hakerem, G. 1976. Evoked potentials in hyperkinetic and normal children under certainty and uncertainty: A placebo and methylphenidate study. Psychophysiology 13:419–428.

Quinn, P. O., and Rapoport, J. L. 1974. Minor physical anomalies and neurologic status in hyperactive boys. Pediatrics 53:742–747.

Rapoport, J. L., Buchsbaum, M. S., Zahn, T. P., Weingartner, H., Ludlow, C., and Mikkelson, E. J. 1978. Dextroamphetamine: Cognitive and behavioral effects in normal prepubertal boys. Science 199:560–563.

Rapoport, J. L., Quinn, P. O., and Lamprecht, F. 1974. Minor physical anomalies and plasma dopamine β-hydroxylase activity in hyperactive boys. Am. J. Psychiatry 131:386–390.

Rapoport, J. L., Quinn, P. O., Scribanu, N., and Murphy, D. L. 1975. Platelet serotonin of hyperactive school age boys. Br. J. Psychiatry 125:138–140.

Riccio, D. C., Rohrbaugh, M., and Hodges, L. A. 1968. Developmental aspects of passive and active avoidance learning in rats. Dev. Psychobiol. 1:108–111.

Robinson, T. E., Vanderwolf, C. H., and Pappas, B. A. 1977. Are the dorsal noradrenergic bundle projections from the locus coeruleus important for neocortical or hippocampal activation? Brain Res. 138:75–98.

Safer, S., and Allen, R. 1976. Hyperactive Children. University Park Press, Baltimore.

Saletu, B., Saletu, M., Simeon, J., Viamontes, G., and Itil, T. 1975. Comparative symptomology and evoked potential studies with d-amphetamine, thioridazine and placebo in hyperkinetic children. Biol. Psychiatry 10:253–275.

Satterfield, J. H., and Braley, B. W. 1977. Evoked potentials and brain maturation in hyperactive and normal children. Electroencephalogr. Clin. Neurophysiol. 43:43–51.

Satterfield, J. H., Cantwell, D., Lesser, L. I., and Podosin, R. L. 1972. Physiological studies of the hyperkinetic child: I. Am. J. Psychiatry 128:1418–1424.

Satterfield, J. H., Cantwell, D., Saul, R., and Yusin, A. 1974. Intelligence, academic achievement and EEG abnormalities in hyperactive children. Am. J. Psychiatry 131:391–395.

Satterfield, J. H., Cantwell, D. P., and Satterfield, B. T. 1974. Pathophysiology of the hyperactive child syndrome. Arch. Gen. Psychiatry 31:839–844.

Satterfield, J. H., and Dawson, M. E. 1971. Electrodermal correlates of hyperactivity in children. Psychophysiology 8:191–197.

Schuckit, M. A., Petrich, J., and Chiles, J. 1978. Hyperactivity: Diagnostic confusion. J. Nerv. Ment. Dis. 166:79–87.

Schwent, V. L., and Hillyard, S. A. 1975. Evoked potential correlates of selective attention with multichannel auditory inputs. Electroencephalogr. Clin. Neurophysiol. 38:131–138.

Shaywitz, B. A. 1976. Minimal brain dysfunction: Dopamine depletion? Science 194:452–453.

Shaywitz, B. A., Yager, R. D., and Klopper, J. H. 1976. Selective brain dopamine depletion in developing rats: An experimental model of minimal brain dysfunction. Science 191:305–308.

Shaywitz, B. A., Klopper, J. H., Yager, R. D., and Gordon, J. W. 1976. Paradoxical response to amphetamine in developing rats treated with 6-hydroxydopamine. Nature 261:153–155.

Shaywitz, B. A., Cohen, D. J., and Bowers, M. B. 1977. CSF monoamine metabolites in children with minimal brain dysfunction: Evidence for alteration of brain dopamine. J. Pediatr. 90:67–71.

Shaywitz, S. E., Cohen, D. J., and Shaywitz, B. A. 1978. The biochemical basis of minimal brain dysfunction. J. Pediatr. 92:179–187.

Shetty, T. 1971a. Alpha rhythms in the hyperkinetic child. Nature 234:476.

Shetty, T. 1971b. Photic responses in hyperkinesis of childhood. Science 174:1356–1357.

Shetty, T., and Chase, T. N. 1976. Central monoamines and hyperkinesis of childhood. Neurology 26:1000–1002.

Silbergeld, E. K., and Goldberg, A. M. 1974. Lead-induced behavioral dysfunction: An animal model of hyperactivity. Exp. Neurol. 42:146–157.

Silbergeld, E. K., and Goldberg, A. M. 1976. Hyperactivity. In A. M. Goldberg, and I. Hanin (eds.), Biology of Cholinergic Function, pp. 619–645. Raven Press, New York.

Snyder, S. H., and Meyerhoff, J. L. 1973. How amphetamine acts in minimal brain dysfunction. Ann. N.Y. Acad. Sci. 205:310–320.

Sobotka, T. J., and Cook, M. P. 1974. Postnatal lead acetate exposure in rats: Possible relation to minimal brain dysfunction. Am. J. Ment. Defic. 79:5–9.

Sobrian, S. K., Weltman, M., and Pappas, B. A. 1975. Neonatal locomotor and long-term behavioral effects of d-amphetamine in the rat. Dev. Psychobiol. 8:241–250.

Spring, C., Greenberg, L., Scott, J., and Hopwood, J. 1974. Electrodermal activity in hyperactive boys who are methylphenidate responders. Psychophysiology 11:436–442.

Sroufe, L. A. 1975. Drug treatment of children with behavior problems. In F. D. Horowitz, E. M. Heatherington, S. Scarr-Salapatek, and G. M. Siegal (eds.), Review of Child Development Research, Vol. 4. University of Chicago Press, Chicago, Ill.

Sroufe, L. A., Sonies, B. C., West, W. D., and Wright, F. S. 1973. Anticipatory heart rate deceleration and reaction time in children with and without referral for learning disability. Child Dev. 44:267–273.

Stein, L. 1978. Reward transmitters: Catecholamines and opioid peptides. In M. A. Lipton, A. DiMascio, and K. F. Killam (eds.), Psychopharmacology: A Generation of Progress, pp. 569–581. Raven Press, New York.

Stevens, J. R., Kuldip, S., and Milstein, V. 1968. Behavior disorders of childhood and the electroencephalogram. Arch. Neurol. 18:160–177.

Stewart, M. A. 1970. Hyperactive children. Sci. Am. 222:94–98.

Tagliomonte, A., Biggio, G., Vargui, L., and Gessa, G. L. 1973. Increase of brain tryptophan and stimulation of serotonin synthesis by salicylate. J. Neurochem. 20:909–912.

Taylor, K. M., and Snyder, S. H. 1970. Amphetamine: Differentiation by *d* and *l* isomers of behavior involving brain norepinephrine and dopamine. Science 168:1487–1489.

Ungerstedt, U. 1974. Brain dopamine neurons and behavior. In F. O. Schmitt and F. G. Worden (eds.), The Neurosciences: Third Study Program, pp. 695–707. The MIT Press, Cambridge, Mass.

Waldrop, M. F., Bell, R. Q., McLaughen, B., and Halverson, C. F. 1978. Newborn minor physical anomalies predict short attention span, peer aggression and impulsivity at age 3. Science 199:563–565.

Wender, P. H. 1969. Platelet-serotonin level in children with "minimal brain dysfunction." Lancet 2:1012.

Wender, P. H. 1971. Minimal Brain Dysfunction in Children. Wiley-Interscience, New York.

Wender, P. H. 1974. Some speculations concerning a possible biochemical basis of minimal brain dysfunction. Life Sci. 14:1605–1621.

Wender, P. H. 1976. The Hyperactive Child—Handbook for Parents. Crown Publishers Inc., New York.

Wender, P. H. 1978. Minimal brain dysfunction: An overview. In M. A. Lipton, A. DiMascio, and K. F. Killan (eds.), Psychopharmacology: A Generation of Progress. Raven Press, New York.

Wender, P. H., Epstein, R. S., Kopin, I. J., and Gordon, E. K. 1971. Urinary monoamine metabolites in children with minimal brain dysfunction. Am. J. Psychiatry 127:1411–1415.

Werry, J. S., and Sprague, R. L. 1970. Hyperactivity. In C. G. Costello (ed.), Symptoms of Psychopathology, p. 397. John Wiley & Sons, Inc., New York.

Wikler, A., Dixon, J. F., and Parker, J. B. 1970. Brain function in problem children and controls. Psychometric, neurological and electrocephalographic comparisons. Am. J. Psychiatry 127:634–645.

Wood, D. R., Reimherr, F. W., Wender, P. H., and Johnson, G. E. 1976. Diagnosis and treatment of minimal brain dysfunction in adults. Arch. Gen. Psychiatry. 33:1453–1460.

Wurtman, R. J., and Fernstrom, J. D. 1975. Control of brain monoamine synthesis by diet and plasma amino acids. Am. J. Clin. Nutr. 28:638–647.

Zahn, T. P., Abate, F., Little, B. C., and Wender, P. H. 1975. Minimal brain dysfunction, stimulant drugs, and autonomic nervous system activity. Arch. Gen. Psychiatry 32:381–387.

Factors Possibly Implicated in Hyperactivity

Feingold's Hypothesis and Hypersensitivity Reactions

Helen Tryphonas

There is increasing evidence that hyperactivity in children is a final common pathway for a variety of etiological factors. Among these are neurological complications following prenatal or perinatal trauma (Minde, Webb, and Sykes, 1968), maternal smoking during pregnancy (Dawson, Nanson, and McWatters, 1976), environmental pollutants, particularly metals such as lead (David, 1974), fluorescent lights (Arehart-Teichel, 1974), familial stress, and genetic transmission (Waldrop and Halverston, 1971). Additional but less well-defined factors believed to contribute to the etiology of hyperactivity include ingestion of artificial food additives such as colors and flavors (Waldrop and Halverston, 1971) and hypersensitivity reactions to a variety of substances (Hall, 1976).

FEINGOLD'S HYPOTHESIS

During the last 3 years much publicity has been attributed to a hypothesis that chemicals added to foods cause adverse behavioral disorders in the pediatric age group. Dr. Ben Feingold, the originator of this hypothesis, made the assertion at the 1973 annual meeting of the American Medical Association that the ingestion of artificial food additives (colors and flavors) and of naturally occurring salicylates in foods results in hyperactivity and learning disabilities in children (Feingold et al., 1973). It is Dr. Feingold's clinical experience that a significant

93

percentage (25%–50%) of children afflicted with behavioral and/or learning problems improve dramatically when given the Kaisar-Permanente diet (K-P diet), which is designed to eliminate all foods containing natural salicylates and artificial colors and flavors from the child's diet. Sufficient improvement to replace drug management has been reported for 75% of the children on the diet (Feingold, 1975a).

Symptoms of hyperactivity, aggression, and impulsiveness are thought to be diminished in the early stages of the diet implementation. This is followed by improvement in motor coordination, manifested by improved writing and drawing, improved speech, and loss of clumsiness. In younger children specific disturbances of perception and cognition are also reported to improve (Feingold, 1975b).

Similar beneficial effects of the K-P diet have been reported from studies conducted in Australia (Cook and Woodhill, 1976; Salzman, 1976). The Cook and Woodhill study included 15 children clinically diagnosed as hyperactive who were instructed to follow the Australian version of Feingold's diet for 9 months. Assessment of progress depended heavily on parental assessments supplemented by classroom and clinical observations. At the end of 9 months, the parents of 10 children indicated that they were "quite certain" and parents of three others were "fairly certain" that: 1) the diet had effected a substantial decrease in the child's hyperactive behavior; and 2) infractions of the diet could cause a reversion to the previous hyperactive behavior patterns. According to the parents' reports, improvement was noticed by others outside the family, such as classroom and remedial teachers.

In the second study (Salzman, 1976), 31 children with behavioral problems (overactivity, sleep problems, lack of concentration, and hyperactivity) were tested for sensitivity to salicylates and artificial colors and flavors by the sublingual provocation method (Hawley and Buckey, 1974). Positive responses included a fall in systolic blood pressure accompanied by an increased pulse rate, a change in pallor, increased perspiration, reduction in activity, skin rashes, and hyperactivity. Eighteen children responded positively to the challenge tests, and fifteen of the 18 followed the elimination diet (Australian version of Feingold's diet) for 4 weeks. A statistically significant improvement was found in scores of impulsiveness, excitability, overactivity, distractibility, and conduct at home following implementation of the elimination diet.

The aforementioned studies offer clinical evidence for the efficiency of the elimination diet in reducing hyperactivity in a substantial number of hyperactive children. There are, however, some variables that have not been considered in these studies, perhaps because of uncontrollable circumstances. In the Australian studies, for example, like those of Feingold, ratings of improvement have been global rather than specific, and objective rating scales (Conners Parent Teacher Rating Scales) were not used. The homogeneity of the sample therefore remains uncertain. Furthermore, the lack of a control group for placebo diet effects, diet order effect, or food intake monitoring makes these studies vulnerable to alternative explanations of the children's "favorable response" to the elimination diet.

Despite the clinical nature of Feingold's claims, the hypothesis has been received favorably and enthusiastically by millions of parents and guardians of hyperactive children and has raised much controversy on the use and safety of artificial food additives. In view of the alarming public anxiety, and the lack of scientifically sound experimental designs to test Feingold's hypothesis, the Nutrition Foundation formed a National Advisory Committee on Hyperkinesis and Food Additives. Scientists with medical, nutrition, and behavioral backgrounds formed this Committee with the aim of reviewing pertinent literature and producing guidelines and suggestions for future research. The Committee produced their first report to the Nutrition Foundation in 1976, with the following conclusions:

1. Studies to date have not shown that hyperkinesis is related to the ingestion of food colors.
2. A significant reduction of hyperactive behaviors when children are placed on the K-P diet has not been experimentally demonstrated.
3. The diet should be used only with competent medical supervision.

A second panel of experts was organized by the Food and Drug Administration in July 1975 (Food and Drug Administration, 1975) to form the Interagency Collaborative Group on Hyperkinesis (ICGH). A preliminary report from the ICGH (Food and Drug Administration, 1976) stated that studies to date "have neither proven nor disproven the hypothesis that a diet free of artificial food colors and flavors reduces the symptoms in a significant number of children with the hyperkinetic behavior syndrome." However, the report further noted that "the evidence taken as a whole is sufficient to merit further investigation into the relationship of diet and the hyperkinetic syndrome" (Food and Drug Administration, 1976).

As a result of these controversial reports, two important studies were designed to test Feingold's hypothesis. These studies are important because hyperactivity was diagnosed in children using objective criteria, and baseline behavioral data were collected during the pretreatment period. Subsequently, approximately one-half of the children, randomly selected, were given the K-P elimination diet for 4 weeks and switched to a placebo diet for an additional 4 weeks. The remaining children received diets in the reverse order.

Fifteen hyperactive children of school age were included in the first study (Conners et al., personal communication). Families of these children were instructed to shop for the appropriate foods themselves and efforts were made to ensure that neither parents nor teachers nor the investigator knew which diet the children were on during the experiment. Parents and teachers observed the children, using Conners' standardized symptom rating scales weekly to monitor changes in the symptoms of the hyperactivity syndrome.

A statistically significant reduction in hyperactivity was found in favor of the K-P diet according to the teachers' ratings, but not according to the parents' ratings. However, a pronounced interaction of diet and diet order was observed on reanalysis of the same data. Thus the observed reduction in hyperactivity was significant only in the group that received the control diet first and the K-P diet second.

A review of the Clinical Global Impression Scores revealed that only one of the 15 children was markedly improved while on the control diet, four children were moderately improved while on the K-P diet, and one child was moderately improved while on the control diet. Therefore, a total of 26% of the children showed improvement while on the K-P diet.

The second major double-blind crossover dietary study (Harley et al., 1977) included 36 school-age and 10 preschool hyperactive boys. Foods were supplied to all of the families on a weekly basis for the duration of the study.

Analysis of behavior ratings by the parents and teachers revealed a diet-related improvement in behavior of the school-age hyperactive children. This was significant in favor of the K-P diet for ratings made by the parents, but teachers rated more children as improved while on the control diet. Of interest and potential significance, however, is the finding that younger children (ages 3–6) showed a greater positive response on the experimental diet as indicated by parents' ratings. All 10 mothers in this group rated their children's behaviors as improved. Similar behavioral improvements were noticed by four of the seven fathers in the same age group.

These studies indicate that there may be a small subgroup of hyperactive children whose behavior is adversely affected by the ingestion of artificial food colors and flavors. However, the investigators noted that this subgroup is either very small or the relationship of diet manipulation to behavioral change is much less dramatic and predictable than has been described in anecdotal reports, or both, and cautioned that it would be hazardous at this point to draw too many conclusions from this experiment, given the small size of the sample and the lack of consistency in the results.

Following observations of these general studies, investigators took a novel approach to testing Feingold's hypothesis. This involved challenge studies with specific groups of food additives. In one such study (Williams et al., 1977), efforts were made to determine the relative therapeutic effectiveness of the diet (K-P) and drug (stimulant) management of hyperactivity in 26 school-age children. All children were stabilized on the K-P diet for one month. Subsequently, these children were randomly assigned to each of the following treatment conditions:

A. Stimulant medication plus modified K-P diet with control cookies
B. Stimulant medication plus modified K-P diet with challenge cookies*
C. Placebo tablets plus modified K-P diet with control cookies
D. Placebo tablets plus modified K-P diet with challenge cookies

Each challenge cookie contained one-half of the total food coloring a person would consume in a regular diet each day. Conners Parent and Teacher Rating Scales were used to measure the effects of the various treatment conditions.

Parents and teachers rated the children as significantly less hyperactive while on stimulant medication alone. However, there were inconsistent findings about the effects of the diet (K-P diet) and the colors. The diet effects in parent ratings were strongest when the children were on medication (that is, drugs plus diet reduced hyperactivity more than drugs alone), and were minimal when the children were on placebo (treatment C). In contrast, the teacher ratings showed minimal effects when the children were on stimulant medication. However, the teacher ratings showed that artificial colors (treatment D) resulted in an increase in hyperactivity if the children did not receive stimulant medication.

This study is indicative of an additive effect of stimulant medication and the elimination diet in reducing hyperactivity in children. It will be interesting to see if this relationship holds given a longer period of time. Since in the present study each treatment combination was implemented

---

* The challenge cookies contained the following artificial food colors: Red nos. 2, 3, and 4; Blue nos. 1 and 2; Yellow nos. 5 and 6; Green no. 3; and Orange B.

for 1 week only, it would be premature to draw any conclusions about long-term effects of the treatments.

In addition, there is some concern with respect to the selection of the hyperactive children. At the conclusion of the study, seven of the 26 children were thought of as not hyperactive by the investigators.

However, the observation that teachers detected a stronger beneficial effect of the Feingold diet than did the parents may be of significance. It is noted that medication and cookies were ingested by the children at breakfast and during lunch. If one assumes a short-term effect of the treatments, then this effect would be more prominent and noticeable during school hours, diminishing substantially by the time children arrive home for parental observation. This postulated short-duration effect of the food colors is strengthened by similar findings in additional experiments conducted elsewhere (Conners et al., 1977).

Preliminary data from two double-blind challenge trials with artificial food colors suggest that performance on a visual-motor tracking task may be impaired after ingestion of challenge material. This impairment was detectable 1 hour after ingestion of cookies containing the colors. Parents were able to detect significant effects after 3 hours following ingestion of the same cookies (Conners et al., 1977).

HYPERSENSITIVITY REACTIONS

Another important parameter that further complicates the interpretation of experimental results pertaining to the K-P diet and hyperactivity is allergy, especially to foods. Allergy, or hypersensitivity, is the term used to denote an increased reactivity of an individual toward a specific substance, and results from prior exposure of the individual to that substance or to a chemically related substance.

Allergies of various types affect 6%–10% of the population. In addition, about 30 % to 40% more show minor allergic manifestations. Humans may develop allergies to a variety of substances, for example, inhalants, drugs (e.g., penicillin, aspirin), and proteins (Rowe, 1931; Criep, 1969), as well as carbohydrates of animal and plant origin. The most common allergenic foods are cow's milk, chicken's eggs, and cereals. Next in order are fish, nuts, spices, and to a lesser extent vegetables and fruits. An individual who is hypersensitive to a food may have symptoms ranging from nasal stuffiness, hives, eczema, rash, migraine headache, nausea, diarrhea, or even a serious attack of asthma, up to anaphylactic shock or even death.

Numerous cases have been reported that suggest an allergic etiology for a variety of neurological and psychiatric manifestations in children. It has been shown, for example, that cerebral edema due to an allergic reaction in the brain tissue or meninges causes migraine (Goltman, 1936) or convulsions typical of the epileptic form (Kennedy, 1931). Others (Rowe, 1931) have reported cases of hypersomnia, insomnia, and various forms of psychic disturbances and have shown, by eliminating and reintroducing the allergen, that these symptoms are due to allergy of the gastrointestinal tract.

Furthermore, allergy has been associated with minimal brain dysfunction (Baldwin, Kittler, and Ramsay, 1968). Twenty children with abnormal electroencephalograms and positive allergy skin tests to inhalants were investigated. Fifteen, or 75%, of the children had positive skin tests to foods. Following inhalant elimination and dietary restriction based on the allergy test results, nine EEGs returned to normal and two others improved. Children were initially tested for psychological abnormalities using the Wechsler, Stanford-Binet, and Merrill-Palmer tests. Seven of the twenty children were found to have normal intelligence but severe learning problems. Following 6 months of inhalant avoidance and dietary restrictions, a significant improvement in school performance was observed. However, children with initial scores lower than normal showed no improvement in academic ability.

A number of other physicians (Clarke, 1950; Randolph, 1950; Crook et al., 1961; Campbell, 1973) have published clinical evidence for an association of allergy to behavioral problems in children. By controlling allergies to foods and, to a lesser degree, to inhalants and chemicals, they were able to eliminate or substantially reduce symptoms of irritability, aggressiveness, hyperactivity, fatigue, anxiety, nervousness, or severe depression in children.

In addition to the foods, a number of hypersensitivity conditions have been reported in recent years by allergists and dermatologists that appear to be related to the ingestion of foods or medicines containing one or more of the artificial food colors (Lockey, 1959). For example, clinical cases of asthma and urticaria caused by orally ingested FD & C Yellow no. 5 (tartrazine) used to coat dexamethasone (Decadron) tablets have been described (Lockey, 1959). Ingestion of tartrazine has also been shown to be the cause of nonthrombocytopenic vascular purpura (Criep, 1971) and Schönlein-Henoch purpura, also known as allergic vasculitis or allergic vascular purpura (Michaëlsson, Petterson, and Juhlin, 1974).

Hypersensitivity reactions have been attributed to other artificial colors in addition to tartrazine. Lockey, using the sublingual provocative tests, reported clinical cases of hypersensitivity to Yellow No. 6, FD & C Red no. 4, Ponceau 3R, Crown Colony green cake coloring (Lockey, 1971), and FD & C Red no. 2 (Lockey, 1977).

It is not known whether the hypersensitivity reactions to colors have an underlying immunological mechanism. Assessment of their immunological potential depends largely on the extent to which these low molecular weight colors bind with serum proteins.

SUMMARY

The syndrome of hyperactivity is complex, and its causes are diverse. The studies conducted to date clearly indicate the potential difficulties in any attempt to test Feingold's hypothesis. The small sample size used in these experiments reduces the significance of all findings and makes the use of statistical analysis extremely difficult. Perhaps the use of inpatients in future projects will eliminate difficulties related to the control of compliance.

Observations implicating allergy, especially to foods, as a cause of hyperactivity are still equivocal. It is not clear, for example, whether allergy is the primary cause of hyperactivity or its presence in some hyperactive children is incidental. Controlled experiments are needed to distinguish between improvement in hyperactivity resulting from implementation of the K-P diet and improvement resulting from elimination from the child's diet of potentially allergenic foods along with the elimination of artificial food additives, as in Feingold's diet.

Finally, a more precise definition of the hyperactivity syndrome, coupled with strict adherence to guidelines set forth by the National Advisory Committee and the ICGH, will undoubtedly produce experimental results conducive to meaningful conclusions.

REFERENCES

Arehart-Teichel, J. 1974. School lights and problem pupils. Sci. News 105:258–259.

Baldwin, D. G., Kittler, F. J., and Ramsay, R. G. 1968. The relationship of allergy to cerebral dysfunction. South. Med. J. 61:1039.

Campbell, M. B. 1973. Neurologic manifestations of allergic disease. Ann. Allergy 31:485–498.

Clarke, J. 1950. The relation of allergy to character problems in children: A survey. Psychoanalyt. Q. 24:21–23.

Conners, C. K., Goyette, C., Petti, T., and Curtis, L. 1977. A challenge test of diet-responsive hyperkinetic children with artificial colors. Preliminary Report.

Conners, C. K., Goyette, C. H., Southwick, D. A., Lees, T. M., and Andrulonis, P. A. 1978. Food additives and hyperkinesis: A controlled double-blind experiment. Personal communication.

Cook, P. S., and Woodhill, F. M. 1976. The Feingold Dietary Treatment of the hyperkinetic syndrome. Med. J. Aust. 2:85–90.

Criep, L. H. 1969. Atopy: General Considerations in Clinical Immunology and Allergy, 2d. ed. Grune & Stratton, New York.

Criep, L. H. 1971. Allergic vascular purpura. J. Allergy Clin. Immunol. 48:7–12.

Crook, W. G., Harrison, W. W., Crawford, S. E., and Emerson, B. S. 1961. Systemic manifestations due to allergy. Pediatrics 27:790.

David, O. J. 1974. Association between lower level lead concentration and hyperactivity in children. Environ. Health Perspect. 7:17–25.

Dawson, R., Nanson, J. L., and McWatters, M. A. 1976. Hyperkinesis and maternal smoking. Can. Psychiat. Assoc. J. 20:183–187.

Feingold, B. F. 1973. Introduction to Clinical Allergy. Charles C Thomas, Springfield, Ill.

Feingold, B. F. 1975a. Why is Your Child Hyperactive? Random House, New York.

Feingold, B. F. 1975b. Hyperkinesis and learning disabilities linked to artificial food flavors and colors. Am. J. Nurs. 75:793–803.

Feingold, B. F., German, D. F., Braham, R. M., and Simmers, E. 1973. Paper presented at the Annual Meeting of the American Medical Association, New York.

Food and Drug Administration. 1975. Proceedings of the September 30, 1975, meeting of Interagency Collaborative Group on Hyperkinesis. U.S. Food and Drug Administration, Washington, D.C.

Food and Drug Administration. 1976. First report of the preliminary findings and recommendations of the Interagency Collaborative Group on Hyperkinesis. U.S. Food and Drug Administration, Washington, D.C.

Goltman, A. M. 1936. The mechanism of migraine. J. Allergy 7:351.

Hall, K. 1976. Allergy of the nervous system: A review. Ann. Allergy 36:49–64.

Harley, T., Ray, R., Tomasi, L., Eichman, P., Matthews, C., Chun, R., and Cleeland, C. 1977. An experimental evaluation of hyperactivity and food additives—Phase 1. Supported by the University of Wisconsin Food Research Institute (Grant #133-9051); data analysis funded by the Department of Health, Education and Welfare (Contract #233-76-2041).

Hawley, C., and Buckey, R. 1976. Food dyes and hyperkinetic children. Academ. Ther. 10:27.

Kennedy, F. 1931. On the nature of fits. Bull. N.Y. Acad. Med. (2nd series) 7:221.

Lockey, S. D. 1959. Allergic reactions due to FD & C Yellow No. 5 Tartrazine and Aniline Dye used as a colouring and identifying agent in various steroids. Ann. Allergy 17:719–721.

Lockey, S. D. 1971. Reactions to hidden agents in foods, beverages and drugs. Ann. Allergy 29:461–466.

Lockey, S. D. 1977. Hypersensitivity to Tartrazine (FD & C Yellow No. 5) and other dyes and additives present in foods and pharmaceutical products. Ann. Allergy 38:206–211.

Michaëlsson, G., Petterson, L., and Juhlin, L. 1974. Purpura caused by food and drug additives. Arch. Dermatol 109:49–52.

Minde, K., Webb, C., and Sykes, D. 1968. Studies on the hyperactive child: VI. Prenatal and perinatal factors associated with hyperactivity. Dev. Med. Child Neurol. 10:355–363.

National Advisory Committee on Hyperkinesis and Food Additives, 1976. Report to the Nutrition Foundation.

Randolph, T. G. 1950. Allergic factors in the etiology of certain mental symptoms. J. Lab. Clin. Med. 36:977.

Rowe, A. H. 1931. Food Allergy: Its Manifestations, Diagnosis and Treatment. Lea & Febiger, Philadelphia.

Rowe, A. H. 1937. Clinical Allergy Due to Foods, Inhalants, Contactants, Fungi, Bacteria and Other Causes. Lea & Febiger, Philadelphia.

Salzman, L. K. 1976. Allergy testing, psychological assessment and dietary treatment of the hyperactive child syndrome. Med. J. Aust. 2:248–251.

Waldrop, M., and Halverston, C. F. 1971. Minor physical anomalies and hyperactive behavior in your children. In J. Hellmuth (ed.), Exceptional Infant, Vol. 2. Brunner/Mazel, New York.

Williams, T. I., Cram, D. M., Tansig, F. T., and Webster, T. 1977. An experimental study of the relative effects of drugs and diet on hyperactive behaviors. Health Care Research Unit, University of Western Ontario. (Unpublished manuscript).

Werry, J. S. 1976. Food additives and hyperactivity. Med. J. Aust. 2:281–283.

Can Hyperactives
Be Identified
in Infancy?

J. L. Rapoport,
P. O. Quinn,
C. Burg,
and
L. Bartley

The aim of this chapter is to survey the prediction of hyperactivity, or minimal brain dysfunction (MBD), in infancy, which is a most ambitious task. An attempt is made to do so using a limited approach, and some general points are presented that are of importance to anyone who addresses the question of prediction from infancy.

In the 1960s Pasamanick and Knobloch (1960) suggested that certain pre- and perinatal risk factors, such as bleeding in pregnancy or low birth weight, showed significant relationships with learning and behavior problems when the child was of school age. That was a historically important study because it came at a time when there was an overemphasis on purely psychological and environmental variables. The Knobloch and Pasamanick work shifted this overemphasis considerably. It had the result, however, of making many workers too enthusiastic in accepting the notion of prediction from pre- and perinatal variables. In Werner's book *The Children of Kauai* (Werner, Bierman, and French, 1971), there is an excellent review of the literature on such prediction that helps to put the early studies into perspective. Some general points emerge when studies of "high risk" newborns are compared.

As reviewed by Werner et al. (1971), it can be seen that when perinatal complications are examined in relation to neurological, perceptual, or developmental measures in the first 3 years of life, some prediction is possible. The studies of Graham et al. (1957, 1962) and

Honzik, Hutchings, and Burnip (1965) found that perinatal complications predicted irritability or emotional withdrawal in infancy (before age 3). The relationships were weak, but they demonstrated that if you look at the children early on (usually before the age that they are likely to have clinical-psychiatric complaints), then you may have some success in predicting problems in infancy from pre- and perinatal risk measures.

If we examine the effects of perinatal complications at school age, however, by looking at children between the ages of 8 and 19, then success in predicting problems is less likely (Werner et al., 1971), and it is only the extreme disabilities, such as mental retardation or physical handicaps, that can be predicted to any significant degree. The first point, then, is that pre- and perinatal measures tend to "wash out" over time.

A second point that emerges from a survey of infant prediction is that univariate analysis is too simplistic to generate useful clinical information. Two epidemiological studies illustrate this point.

The first study is the Kauai study (Werner et al., 1971), in which more than 1000 pregnancies were followed for almost two decades (Werner et al., 1971; Werner and Smith, 1977). Werner's group understandably chose to work on the island of Kauai (it is a very good place for a long-term follow-up study from the point of view of both the researchers and the relatively stable island population).

The Werner group was able to look at their population, prospectively, in a complex way. They began with 3000 pregnancies and followed over 1000 of these infants to age 18. Because of their complete planning and follow-up, they had data not only on school behavior, but on the home support system as well. In addition, on the island of Kauai public prenatal medical health care was excellent and virtually independent of socioeconomic status.

When severity of perinatal stress was examined alone in relation to school achievement or hyperkinetic behavior disorders at age 10, there were no significant relationships except for mental retardation or significant physical handicaps. When social variables were also used in the analysis, however, powerful relationships emerged between severity of perinatal stress and behavioral measures for those with lower socioeconomic status, as well as for those with below-average emotional support in the home. This point may seem evident to some; nevertheless, at clinical conferences we often refer to, for example, a child's having a low birth weight as being "clear" evidence that this is an "organic" child or that some other clinical phenomena could have been predicted early on if someone had noted the mother's difficulties in pregnancy.

For completeness, it should be noted that the hyperkinetic syndrome per se was not particularly well predicted in the Kauai study by any social measure except "educational stimulation" of the home. On the other hand, school achievement and "emotional problems" as a whole were predicted at age 10 when social factors were taken into consideration. The point is that there is a group of vulnerable children whose environment may not make up for insults during the prenatal period.

The second epidemiological study is the Collaborative Project of the National Institute of Neurologic Diseases and Stroke (NINCDS), in which over 50,000 pregnancies were followed at 12 affiliated hospital centers, from the time of the mother's first missed period until the child reached the age of 7. Both pre- and perinatal data were collected prospectively, as well as developmental measures when the child was ages 1, 4, and 7. Academic and neurological testing was done, with rating of behavior noted by the psychologist during testing. The study lacked behavior rating by teachers and, although there were socioeconomic measures, the Collaborative Project was not able to include measures of emotional support or of educational stimulation in the home. Dr. Paul Nichols (1976) of NINCDS has examined the scores for the Academic, Neurological, and Behavioral Measures for over 30,000 of these children of normal intelligence who were followed until age 7. Dr. Nichols obtained factor scores for academic achievement, hyperactivity, neurological problems, and immaturity. These measures were all from clinic ratings alone. Nichols did not have the complete data that the Kauai group had; however, since the measures were coordinated between the different centers, he was able to establish scores for each child on the factors that people in a general way refer to as the hyperactivity syndrome, or MBD. He found that 6% of his sample could be considered as hyperactive according to their scores on these factors.

Nichols examined behavioral, cognitive, perceptual, motor, academic achievement, and neurological measures for the group as established at the age 7 exam. Using this large cohort, he predictably found some associations between behavioral and neurological scores with (interestingly enough) the weakest association between the cognitive and the neurological measures. The relation of the prenatal variables to the 7-year exam scores was examined and there were some predictive relationships between measures. For example, if the mother smoked three packs of cigarettes or more per day, or if proteinuria was present during pregnancy, then there was some relationship to hyperactivity, low academic achievement, or neurologic soft signs. However, any suspected abnormality in the neonatal period only increased the likelihood of MBD at age 7 by about 5%. This is important to keep in mind, because clinicians are regularly asked to make some clinical formulation of a large amount of data (including both obstetrical and socioeconomic facts) about a particular child. One needs to remember, when evaluating a child from a grossly deprived background who has low emotional support and low educational stimulation, that these social factors have a more powerful causative influence than the mother's smoking or even bleeding during pregnancy. Nichols (1976) has shown that prenatal predictors increase the likelihood of MBD from 2% to 5%, whereas evidence from the Kauai study shows that the social and emotional support system to the child may increase the likelihood of pathology by 200%–400%!

Now the background review explains why we have not pursued pre- and perinatal problems per se in relation to childhood psychopathology, a second question is whether it will be worthwhile to identify behavior problems in infancy; that is, will it be of practical value to clinicians to identify behavior problems in the first 3 years of life? There is more positive and, I think, more interesting data in this area.

A few studies have suggested that it is indeed worthwhile to identify infants (that is, preschoolers and toddlers) who have behavior problems. In a study in 1961, Wolff followed up 43 preschool children who were first seen at a child guidance clinic at age 3. When seen 3 to 6 years after clinic contact, there was generally a continuity of symptoms, with worse outcomes for boys than for girls. Although Wolff was not studying hyperactivity in particular, her clinic population presented chiefly with the behaviors associated with the hyperactivity syndrome, such as "overactivity" and tantrums. In a Canadian study from Montreal, Campbell et al. (1977) followed up 20 hyperactive children who had been studied in a research nursery school at age 4. When these children were 6½ years old, hyperactivity was still reported. They still had more behavior problems than controls; moreover, ratings of extreme activity in the nursery school had some prediction within the samples—that is, extremely hyperactive children did not do as well as the moderately hyperactive ones. These preschool studies, therefore, show that the symptoms of hyperactivity (unlike symptoms of fearfulness and phobias) have moderate predictivity for middle childhood. Research into infant and toddler behavioral disturbances therefore does seem clinically worthwhile.

Our interest in infant studies has developed over the past few years. In 1974, as part of an outpatient drug study of hyperactivity, (Rapoport et al., 1974), we assembled a large number of relatively homogeneous middle-class boys, ages 6 to 12 and of normal intelligence, with the presenting complaint of "hyperactivity." One measure of great interest to us was that of minor physical anomalies of the face, head, hands, and feet. These anomalies are listed in Table 1.

These anomalies attracted our interest from several viewpoints. First, they are found to a greater extent in association with central nervous system disease than with anomalous development of other systems. Smith and Bostian (1964) showed that children with idiopathic mental retardation were more likely to have three or more minor anomalies than were a group of patients with cleft lip or palate or ventricular septal defect. Forty-two percent of children with mental retardation, but only ten percent of those with cleft palate, for example, had three or more anomalies. None of the control children had more than two anomalies.

Goldfarb (1967) examined a group of "schizophrenic" children for some of these anomalies and found a high incidence in association with schizophrenic as compared with normal children. In a study with normal first-grade children, Rosenberg and Weller (1973) looked at these minor physical anomalies early in the school year. At the end of the academic year, they were able to relate promotion to the second grade to the total and weighted scores for these anomalies. The Rosenberg and Weller finding was for a group with normal intelligence, and supported a relationship between anomaly scores and behavior that was independent of IQ.

The particular anomalies, shown in Table 1, are formed in the early fetal development (Smith, 1970). They are known to be influenced both by genetic factors and by a variety of toxic substances, as evidenced by the fact that several of the anomalies are present in the fetal alcohol syndrome.

Minor anomaly scores were obtained for the group of 80 boys at the beginning of their clinical evaluation (Quinn and Rapoport, 1974); there was a positive association between the teacher's ratings of hyperactivity and anomaly scores. There was no significant association with other measures of "organicity"; that is, an abnormal EEG or the number of neurological soft signs did not correlate with the anomaly scores.

We had also obtained data as to the age of onset of hyperactivity. There are "early" hyperactives, those whose parents tell you that their child was different and difficult in infancy. They had often sought help from their pediatrician before the child was 1 year old. There is also a group of parents, in contrast to these, who say that they were surprised when the teacher complains that their child was disruptive in the

Table 1.   Anomalies and scoring weights for obtaining the Minor Physical
Anomaly Score (Quinn and Rapoport, 1974)

Anomaly	Scoring weights
Head	
Head circumference	
> 1.5 SD	2
1 to 1.5 SD	1
"Electric" hair	
very fine hair that won't comb down	2
fine hair that is soon awry after combing	1
Two or more whorls	0
Eyes	
Epicanthus: where upper and lower lids join at the nose, point of union is	
deeply covered	2
partly covered	1
Hypertelorism: approximate distance between tear ducts	
1.5 SD	2
1.25 to 1.5 SD	1
Ears	
Low-set: bottom of ears in line with	
mouth (or lower)	2
area between mouth and nose	1
Adherent lobes: lower edges of ears extend	
upward and back toward crown of head	2
straight back toward rear of neck	1
Malformed	1
Asymmetrical	1
Soft and pliable	0
Mouth	
High palate	
roof of mouth steepled	2
roof of mouth moderately high	1
Furrowed tongue	1
Smooth/rough spots on tongue	0
Hands	
Fifth finger	
markedly curved inward toward other fingers	2
slightly curved inward toward other fingers	1
Single transverse palmar crease	1
Index finger longer than middle finger	0
Feet	
Third toe	
definitely longer than second toe	2
appears equal in length to second toe	1
Partial syndactyly of two middle toes	1
Gap between first and second toe (approximately ¼ inch)	1

classroom. (Our direct observations in the classroom, by the way, did not help us to distinguish these two groups; we were impressed with how accurate the teacher's reports were for both populations.) "High" anomaly children were much more likely to have been considered a "problem," as shown in Table 2, before the age of 3. The clinical history was not taken by the person who obtained the anomaly score. Because of this powerful association with early onset of problems, we felt we had an entré into infant prediction of hyperactivity. Other infant behaviors, such as head banging (a common problem in infancy), also correlated with the anomaly score.

We then looked at the child's anomaly score in relation to family history of hyperactivity as well as to obstetrical risk factors. We were interested in both genetic and obstetrical features, since the minor anatomical deviations have been related to both types of adverse influences. We found a statistically significant difference between those children who had a family history of hyperactivity and those without, as reported elsewhere (Quinn and Rapoport, 1974; Rapoport and Quinn, 1975). Obstetrical complications showed an even more striking relationship to anomaly score that was particularly strong for the severe complications.

In summary, anomaly scores related to background genetic and toxic factors that would be expected in terms of what is known about the formation of these anomalies. In addition, these anomalies can be measured at birth, and so could be used as part of a newborn screening study. We were convinced that we had a subgroup of hyperactive children that might be identified early in life. A stepwise discriminant function analysis (shown in Table 3) that was based on age of onset, plasma dopamine-β-hydroxylase (DBH) level, paternal history, and obstetrical history supported the notion of such a subgroup.

Another study examined the generality of high anomaly scores to other deviant patient groups (Steg and Rapoport, 1975). An interrater reliability of 0.90 between two different raters was obtained for anomaly scoring. Children from the pediatric ward (excluding those with neu-

Table 2.   Weighted stigmata score and age of onset of hyperactivity for low and high stigmata patients[a]

	Seen as problems	
Stigmata score	Before age 3	After age 3
5 or more	21	3
Less than 5	20	37

[a] $N = 81$; $\chi^2 = 16.50$; $p < 0.001$.

Table 3. Classification outcome table—stepwise linear discriminant function based on age of onset, plasma dopamine-β-hydroxylase, paternal hitory, and obstetrical history[a]

Stigmata	"Computer low"	"Computer high"
High (6–10); $N = 18$	5	13
Low (0–3); $N = 40$)	39	1

[a] $\chi^2 = 32.98; p < .001$.

rologic problems) and children from the Georgetown Hospital Child Guidance Clinic had low scores, whereas a group of unsocialized, aggressive, conduct-disordered children and a group of learning-disabled children were higher. This was a statistical association, however, and there were false positives and false negatives. Nevertheless, the study indicated that a variety of disabilities might be identified in part on the basis of an early screening.

Having decided to do a newborn study, we then had to concern ourselves with behavioral measurement in infancy. In our study (Quinn et al., 1977), we were able to screen 933 infants from the newborn nursery who were on the private service at Georgetown University Hospital over a 14-month period. We were able to obtain both "high" and "low" anomaly infants; the distribution of anomaly scores for the group is shown in Table 4.

In planning our follow-up behavioral measures, we included a standard developmental test as well as checklist and interview ratings of temperament and behavior. After the screening, we followed the top and bottom 8% (approximately) of the samples with respect to anomaly score

Table 4. Frequency (f) and percentage (%) of weighted scores for total newborn screening sample ($N = 933$)[a]

		Weighted Score								
		0	1	2	3	4	5	6	7	8	9
Males ($N = 423$)	f	5	59	155	122	110	23	11	3	4	
	%	1	12	31	24	22	5	2	0.6	0.8	
Females ($N = 441$)	f	8	37	148	94	104	24	16	8	1	1
	%	2	8	33	21	23	5	3	2	0.2	0.2
Total sample ($N = 933$)	f	13	96	303	216	214	47	27	11	5	1
	%	1.3	10	32	23	23	5	3	1.5	0.5	0.1

[a] From Quinn et al., 1977.

prospectively. Interviewers and testers have seen the children yearly and our testing staff has remained blind for anomaly score.

Behavioral measurement in infancy is crude. However, we did have the landmark work of Chess and co-workers (1962) studying temperament in infancy as a guide. Chess and Thomas identified some "unfavorable" characteristics of infant temperament that could be elicited from interviews if mothers were asked about specific behaviors of the infant in specific situations, such as how the child behaved when he had to sleep in a new place, get a shot at the doctor's office, ran a fever, tried new foods, etc. General dimensions of temperament were identified, such as intensity, rhythmicity, approach, and mood. Chess and Thomas showed that some later prediction was possible from these early temperamental characteristics (Rutter et al., 1964). Carey has developed a 70-item questionnaire that could be scored using the dimensions of rhythmicity, approach, withdrawal, mood, and so on that parents can complete. Carey had used this temperament questionnaire in his pediatric practice to predict later events such as learning problems, night waking, colic, and so on (Carey, 1970, 1973). Carey's questionnaires were completed for all study infants at ages 6 months and 1 year. In addition to temperament scales, a pediatric interview with the parents about specific problems of allergies, night waking, and so on was carried out. At ages 2 and 3, we also used the interview schedule developed by Richman, Stevenson, and Graham (1975) for their study of preschool behavioral problems. Richman had developed this interview for 3-year-olds, and we had to adapt it for use with 2-year-olds. Interrater reliabilities have been high (above 0.90) for both 2- and 3-year-old interviews.

At age 6 months, there were some positive correlations between individual items of "difficult temperament" and the newborn plasma concentration of the enzyme dopamine-β-hydroxylase (DBH), as has been reported elsewhere (Rapoport et al., 1977). Infants higher on DBH were more likely to be unsociable, more negative, and more tense.

We obtained our own norms for 1-year-olds on the Carey temperament questionnaire, which had been standardized only for 4- to 8-month-old infants. Positive findings at age 1 and age 2 for our sample are summarized in Table 5.

In general, "difficult" infants are those considered to be high in activity and intensity, low in rhythmicity, adaptability, and approach, and low in threshold and moods. As shown in Table 5, when we examined the infants' behaviors at age 1, we found that, for males, high anomaly 1-year-olds were considered more difficult on three temperament measures as well as on the pediatric interview. We were reassured to find some significant relationship between activity as obtained in the pediatric interview and that obtained by direct observations during Bailey testing at age 1 year, even though these correlations were low. As seen, we do not have a clearly "distractible," as opposed to "intense negative," infant. It seems that there is a fairly close association between these traits among our "difficult" babies.

When obstetrical difficulties were examined in relation to 1-year behavior, we found a significant relation between obstetrical history and irritability only for the high anomaly group (Quinn et al., 1977). This suggests that within different subgroups of infants there will be different causative factors. Significant differences between low and high anomaly groups at age 2 are shown in Table 5. Again, for males, high anomaly infants are less cooperative and more irritable, and high anomaly females have a more negative emotional tone.

The data are not yet complete for the 3-year-old measure, since we have only seen 75 of our 123 patients for 3-year follow-up at this time. Our preliminary data are shown in Table 6: high anomaly 3-year-olds tended to have a higher total behavior score on the Richman and Graham interview (a score of 5.3 as opposed to the high anomaly group having a score of 6.5). Teacher ratings for those who attended preschool, using the Bell-Waldrop preschool scale (Bell, Waldrop and Weller, 1972), suggest that high anomaly females are more difficult than low anomaly

Table 5. Chi-square values for measures distinguishing high (≥ 5) and low (≤ 3) anomaly infants at 1- and 2-year follow-up

Age	Variable	Males			Females		
		χ^2	df	p	χ^2	df	p
1 year	Pediatric interview						
	Irritability	7.07	2	0.03			
	Temperament scale						
	Adaptability	5.93	1	0.02			
	Threshold	5.82	1	0.02			
	Mood	4.80	1	0.03			
	Activity[a]				18.05	6	0.005
	Approach				4.46	1	0.03
2 years	Psychologist rating						
	Cooperativeness	11.05	5	0.05			
	Emotional tone				12.05	5	0.05
	Parent interview						
	Irritability	8.23	2	0.01			
	Night waking	6.88	2	0.03			

[a] High anomaly females are less active.

Table 6. Significant differences between low and high anomaly 3-year-olds, based on newborn anomaly score

| | Teacher ratings | | | |
	Inability to delay	Nomadic play	Vacant staring	Richman Behavior Problem Score
Females				
Low anomaly (N = 12)	2.08 (2.06)	3.75 (1.21)	1.33 (0.77)	
High anomaly (N = 10)	4.08 (3.32)	5.00 (1.88)	3.10 (1.88)	
t	2.13	1.89	2.18	
p	0.02	0.05	0.02	
Low anomaly (N = 20)				4.75 (2.46)
High anomaly (N = 15)				6.33 (2.66)
t				1.83
p				0.05
Males and females				
Low anomaly (N = 41)				5.34 (2.23)
High anomaly (N = 34)				6.55 (2.39)
t				2.34
p				0.01

females. More females were enrolled in preschool than males at age 3, so this may be an artifact of sampling.

In summary, we are encouraged by these positive findings indicating that some differences may be identifiable in infancy between low anomaly and high anomaly preschool children. We do not feel that a measure of anomalies by itself will prove clinically useful. Werner has already shown that measures of educational stimulation and emotional support in the home must be included in order for a predictive study to have clinical usefulness. Our comparisons are statistically significant, but numerically small.

Because the number of false positives (that is, high anomaly infants who appear problem free) that we obtain is large, there is the danger of a "self-fulfilling prophecy"—early identification by this method might do more harm than good. The *combination* of temperament, background factors, and anomalies may prove helpful in other studies in predicting infant problems; the association of anomalies with "difficult" infant temperament supports the idea of congenital contributors to behavior.

REFERENCES

Bell, R., Waldrop, M., and Weller, G. 1972. A rating system for the assessment of hyperactive and withdrawn children in preschool samples. Am. J. Orthopsychiatry 42:23–34.

Campbell, S., Schleitter, M., Weiss, G., and Perlman, T. 1977. A two-year follow-up of hyperactive preschoolers. Am. J. Orthopsychiatry 47:149–162.

Carey, W. 1970. A simplified method for measuring infant temperament. J. Pediatr. 77:188–194.

Carey, W. 1973. Measurement of infant temperament in pediatric practice. In J. C. Westman (ed.), Individual Differences in Children. John Wiley & Sons, Inc., New York.

Chess, S., Hertzig, M., Birch, H., and Thomas, A. 1962. Methodology of adaptive functions of the preschool child. J. Am. Acad. Child Psychiatry 1:236–245.

Goldfarb, W. 1967. Factors in the development of schizophrenia. In J. Romano (ed.), The Origins of Schizophrenia. Exerpta Medica, New York.

Graham, F., Caldwell, B., Ernhart, C., Pennoyer, M., and Hartmen, A. 1957. Anoxia as a significant perinatal experience: A critique. J. Pediatr. 50:556–569.

Graham, F., Ernhart, C., Thurston, D., and Carft, M. 1962. Development three years after perinatal anoxia and other potentially damaging newborn experiences. Psychol. Monogr. (Serial 522) 76:3.

Honzik, M., Hutchings, J., and Burnip, S. R. 1965. Birth record assessment and test performance at eight months. Am. J. Dis. Child. 109:416–426.

Nichols, P. 1976. Minimal brain dysfunction: Associations with perinatal complications. Paper presnted at the Society for Research in Child Development, New Orleans, March, 1976.

Pasamanick, B., and Knobloch, H. 1960. Brain damage and reproductive casualty. Am. J. Orthopsychiatry 30:298–305.

Quinn, P. Q., and Rapoport, J. 1974. Minor physical anomalies and neurologic status in hyperactive boys. Pediatrics 53:742–747.

Quinn, P., Renfield, M., Burg, C., and Rapoport, J. 1977. Minor physical anomalies. A newborn screening and 1-year follow-up. J. Am. Acad. Child Psychiatry 16:662–669.

Rapoport, J., Prandon, C., Renfield, M., Lake, C. R., and Ziegler, M. 1977. Newborn dopamine-β-hydroxylase, minor physical anomalies and infant temperament. Am. J. Psychiatry 134:676–679.

Rapoport, J., Quinn, P., Bradbord, G., Riddle, D., and Brooks, E. 1974. Imipramine and methylphenidate treatment of hyperactive boys. Arch. Gen. Psychiatry 30:789–796.

Rapoport, J., and Quinn, P. 1975. Minor physical anomalies (stigmata) and early developmental deviation: A major biologic subgroup of hyperactive children. Int. J. Ment. Health 4:29–44.

Richman, N., Stevenson, J., and Graham, P. 1975. Prevalance of behavior problems in 3 year old children: An epidemiological study in a London borough. J. Child Psychol. Psychiatry 16:272–287.

Rosenberg, J., and Weller, G. 1973. Minor physical anomalies and academic performance in young school children. Dev. Med. Child Neurol. 13:131–135.

Rutter, M., Birch, H., Thomas, A., and Chess, S. 1964. Temperamental characteristics in infancy and the later development of behavioral disorders. Br. J. Psychiatry 110:651–661.

Smith, D. 1970. Recognizable patterns of human malformation. In A. J. Schaffer (ed.), Major Problems in Clinical Pediatrics. W. B. Saunders Company, Philadelphia.

Smith, D., and Bostian, K. 1964. Congenital anomalies associated with idiopathic mental retardation. J. Pediatr. 65:189–196.

Steg, J., and Rapoport, J. 1975. Minor physical anomalies in normal, neurotic, learning disabled and hyperactive children. J. Autism Child. Schizophr. 5:299–307.

Werner, E., Bierman, J., and French, F. 1971. The Children of Kauai. University of Hawaii Press, Honolulu.

Werner, E., and Smith, R. 1977. Kauai's Children Come of Age. University of Hawaii Press, Honolulu.

Wolff, S. 1961. Symptomatology and outcome of preschool children with behavior disorders attending a child guidance clinic. J. Child Psychol. Psychiatry 5:269–276.

Discussion of "Can Hyperactives be Identified in Infancy"

Marcel Kinsbourne

We have two issues to learn about from Dr. Rapoport's approach. One is the issue of etiology—the role of genetic factors in the origin of target behaviors—and the other is the practical issue of predicting children's difficulties on the basis of early findings in general and stigmata in particular.

Unpromising as it may seem to add up miscellaneous anomalies that each score 1 and so are supposedly of equal importance, it is remarkable that one gets significant correlations at all, and no one could complain if they are low. It would have been unusual had they been high. Two points of detail arise. First, I think that an item analysis of specific anomalies such as hydrocephaly or microcephaly might reveal that some characteristics are more predictive than others. The other thing that comes to mind is that some of these anomalies had to do with facial features, whereas others involve more covered places like the toes or the molars. Obviously physical attractiveness is a determinant of how adults and children react to children. One wonders if any of these children had low set ears and crinkly eyelids and just didn't look too great to their parents. Their parents might then have treated them differentially, thus setting up behavior comparable to the temperaments that you are looking for. It would be good to know whether the predictive value of nonvisible anomalies are as great as those of the visible ones.

It was not clear to me from your presentation, but I take it that you partialled out IQ and the relationship held. The impressive relationship between mental retardation and anomalies would of course be the first thing to partial out. The other striking thing is that everything that seemed to correlate significantly (with one exception) could well be genetic rather than related to obstetric complications. Does the tendency toward obstetric complication correlate with hyperactivity in fathers? Is a tendency to complication itself genetically determined in these children? We might either have two contributions to the anomaly score—one genetic and the other obstetric complications—or there might be one antecedent cause only and obstetric complications might not be causative but correlated.

When we have weak correlations, obviously we have to worry primarily about our sampling. If we can only predict 5% of the variance on, say, irritability or activity level from some stable score like the anomaly score, that may be because the relationship is that weak, or because the definition of the temperament was indefinite. One need not necessarily accept that the anomaly score is never going to have more predictive value. Perhaps a refinement of the characterization of the behaviors would purify the relationships.

According to Buss and Plomin (1975), there are four heritable temperaments—activity level, emotionality, sociability, and impulsivity. How do these four temperaments feed into an irritability score? Obviously emotionality would be likely to generate an irritable response to stimulation; impulsivity might be seen to do so also. Low sociability might cause the kind of withdrawal that you note in your female subjects, and of course activity level itself is relevant to restless irritability. We have here four orthogonal variables, and yet all of them could contribute somewhat to your samples of children rated irritable at age 1.

The problem is that you have personality extremes that of course are likely to yield behavioral deviances later, because extremes in relation to any human norm put the person into a relatively maladaptive situation. However, there may be extremes of more than one personality trait, so you may have children in the middle and children at either end of several personality dimensions. In addition, one can be irritable either because one is of irritable temperament, or because one itches or has indigestion. If a child is allergic and feels lousy, he might seem irritable without that being his temperament. I believe you have looked at allergies as one of your variables and did not find correlations. However, we also know as pediatricians that, in particular, the gastrointestinal allergies are not necessarily very well known to parents and others when the child is only 1 year old. Many of these are missed until later. As is often the case in work like this, significant correlations are significant, and insignificant ones merely leave you where you were before you asked the question.

The kinds of questions we ask about our hyperactives in the first year have to do with activity, with sleep patterns, and with colicky behavior. The answers we get are variable. As you pointed out, there are indeed clinically two groups: those parents who say this was a terrible child for the following reasons, and the others who say that the child was normal until a certain age. Now, we as clinicians don't know whether this is reality or parental obliviousness in the case of the second group and I think the finding that you mentioned to us about the difference in anomaly score between the children who were detected early and those who were not is very important. It suggests that, when we get a history stating that hyperactivity wasn't noticed until age 2, 3, or 4, this represents a reality rather than false reporting. That in itself has some implications. Maybe these children are hyperactive for a different reason, be it psychogenic or allergic. Sleep patterns did correlate, and that is interesting. Activity level as such is difficult because, as we agreed earlier, high versus low activity is actually irrelevant to our topic of hyperactivity (paradoxical though it may sound because of the mistaken name for the entity). However, a high activity level and high impulsivity might interact to cause problem behavior. With respect to colic, the baby that is stiff and tense gobbles its food and spits up, and again we are at a loss, because we lack direct observational data. The information is based on reports to doctors. Are these babies in fact overactive and greedy, and do they swallow air with their food and then burp (as we are taught in medical school), or do they have intestinal allergies, or is "colic" a rationalization for generally tense behavior, which happens to be most often noted at those times when the parent most commonly interacts with the baby—the feeding times? When I was sufficiently unspecialized in pediatrics to worry along with mothers who had trouble feeding their babies, I had the mothers put some phenobarbital into the bottle. The mothers came back after two weeks saying almost every time that I had cured the disease. This raises a curious issue. As we heard earlier in the seminar, barbiturates make hyperactivity worse. If colicky behavior were due to hyperactivity, the child should have been made worse by the phenobarbital (if the responsivity in infancy is the same as later). This is a bundle of ifs that leads into the question, what is the response of normal infants with even temperaments to sedatives and stimulants in infancy? Now, we are unlikely to give amphetamine to little babies, but barbiturates are used therapeutically both in the way I've described and for epilepsy. We might learn a lot by noting the response of a child's behavior to those agents given for medical reasons, and find out whether in fact in infancy as in older kids a subset of them become behaviorally more difficult to manage. These might then be considered to be at risk for hyperactivity in later life. A further point about irritability relates to what was discussed earlier in the seminar. We could think of an anxious child as being irritable. We were commenting that Dr. Kløve made a wise move in excluding anxious children from his sample. Who are these irritables? If they are going to be hyperactive, are they going to be "favorable responders" to stimulants who are not anxious or "adverse responders" who are? If we are predicting hyperactivity, which type are we predicting?

Now for the point about the social and emotional support. Again we may ask some questions. There always is a cause and effect issue. Did the inadequate social-emotional support contribute to the child's problem or vice versa? Methodological refinements such as checking social-emotional support given to a child's siblings rather than to the child himself, or prevalent in the family before the child's birth, will help to determine cause and effect. That stricture apart, there does seem to be growing support for the view that when children have temperamental extremes these may not necessarily get them into trouble if the support systems are sound, but these will be the children who react adversely to any environmental stresses.

In conclusion, a few comments need to be made about "state of the art" statements. If we don't understand a problem, we get together and pool our knowledge of it. Then we make a statement that says that we don't understand this problem, but the state of the art is that the following information is the answer to the problem (which we don't understand). We then can legitimately express our ignorance in the form of a definite opinion. With respect to your work, I don't know how high a percentage of the variance you are able to predict. Maybe it is zero for reasons that we have discussed, or maybe it is much more for reasons that we have discussed. I do know that your work in progress is of great interest and we hope to hear more about it.

REFERENCES

Buss, A., and Plomin, R. 1975. A Temperament Theory of Development. Wiley-Interscience, New York.

The Hyperkinetic Syndrome

Criteria for Diagnosis

Hallgrim Kløve
and
Kjell Hole

In a recent review of stimulant drug research with hyperactive children, Barkley (1977) concluded that a characteristic trait of research on hyperactive children is the great variability in the results. Based on a survey of the literature, no definite conclusions can be drawn with regard to incidence of hyperactivity, effectiveness of treatment, psychophysiological response patterns, effects of central nervous system stimulants on psychological functions, and the prognosis of hyperactive children, both treated and untreated. The emphasis of Barkley's review was the necessity to focus on the problems related to criteria for diagnostic classification of children with hyperactive behavior disorders. Without appropriate classification, research results are often meaningless. Two of the factors that require better definition are the view on etiology (which has been rather undifferentiated) and the issue of prior treatment. As far as etiology is concerned, evidence indicates that, although these children behaviorally may have many traits in common, etiologically we are working with a highly diversified group. As for the issue of naïve subjects, it is rather common for hyperactive patients to have been subjected to various kinds of psychological and pharmacological treatment over a long period of time. It is important that researchers know a patient's status in this respect and take it into account. These two factors are only indicative of the many problems present in hyperactivity studies that usually render the results inconclusive.

This study has been supported by the Norwegian Research Council for Science and Humanities.

The hyperactive behavior syndrome as a rule refers to a behavioral description, and it is reasonable to assume that many different causative factors may be operating both singly and in combination to produce hyperactive behavior. This paper addresses itself in particular to the problem of identifying those children in whom a positive effect on behavior may be obtained by using drugs that stimulate the central nervous system (CNS). Barkley's review of the literature, as well as clinical experience, agrees that not all hyperactive children will benefit from the use of such drugs, and an important contribution must be to identify those children in whom they are effective in attenuating symptoms.

Bradley's (1937) observation that dextroamphetamine had a positive effect on undesirable behavior, and a large number of subsequent studies on the effects of stimulant drugs, have resulted in psychologists turning their interest toward psychophysiological research in an attempt to better understand both the pathophysiology and psychopharmacology of hyperkinetic behavior.

The present study is based on two hypotheses:

1. Since in some patients hyperactive behavior improves with the administration of stimulant drugs, the drug is most likely acting on a hypoactive central nervous system. In other words, the idea of a "paradoxical effect" of the centrally stimulating drugs is rejected. It is felt that a theoretical basis for this concept has never been demonstrated and the use of the "paradoxical effect" concept has developed as a result of lack of understanding of the pharmacological action of stimulant drugs in these patients.

2. If stimulant drugs are acting on a hypofunctional nervous system, there ought to be independent evidence supporting the hypothesis of a dysfunctional nervous system. With this in mind, the developmental history of the patients in this study has been analyzed in detail, with the idea of revealing possible deviations in early development.

THE AROUSAL CONCEPT

Since this study addresses itself to problems associated with disturbances in nervous system reactivity and defects in central activating mechanisms, it is necessary to discuss the concept of arousal briefly. Arousal is a rather vaguely defined concept and is often used synonymously with other terms such as activation, awakeness, emotions, and drive (Eysenck, 1970). In general, one could consider arousal as an "intensity dimension" of behavior (Duffy, 1962), and in a neurological context it may represent the degree of cortical activation. In the present context, the concept will be used in the sense that it is related to the degree of awakeness of an organism. One could conceive that the degree of awakeness varies along a dimension from deep sleep or pathological coma on the one end to a hyperaroused state of emotional and cognitive chaos or panic on the other end. An organism's normal arousal level will be found some place between these extremes. Luria (1973) maintained that the general arousal level is dependent on several factors, such as sensory input, metabolic processes, and cortical functioning. In order to function normally and adequately it is necessary that the organism be at an optimal arousal level. Malmo (1959) has demonstrated that the relationship between achievement level and arousal can be described as an inverse curve where both very low and very high arousal levels result in impairment of functioning and achievement. Attention, concentration, cognition, impulse control, and emotional control are disrupted by either high or low extremes of arousal.

Behaviorally, the hyperactive child appears to be in a condition of disordered arousal. However, one must determine whether the hyperactive child will be found on the high end or the low end of the physiological arousal continuum.

This interesting relationship between stimulant drugs and arousal level, coupled with the conceptualization of arousal by Moruzzi and Magoun (1949), has resulted in psychologists' attention being turned toward psychophysiological reaction patterns in hyperactive children. Studies by Boydstun et al. (1968) and Satterfield and Dawson (1971) do indeed suggest that hyperactive children are hypoactive from a CNS reactivity point of view. Satterfield and Dawson found that hyperactive children had a higher skin resistance level and fewer spontaneous skin resistance responses than control children. Both skin resistance levels and the spontaneous skin resistance changes were considered as reliable indicators of general arousal level. These results then indicated that hyperactive children are in a state of low central nervous system arousal as compared with normal children. Satterfield and Dawson formulated, based on this hypothesis, the idea that the high motor activity represents one way for these children to achieve an increased arousal level through a self-induced increase in sensory stimulation. Research results, in general, however, do not give such a clear picture of the dynamics of hyperactivity. In a later publication concerned with the autonomic response pattern of hyperactive children, Satterfield et al. (1974)

obtained results that on many points were contradictory to the 1971 findings. In fact, a review of the present evidence suggests that it is not appropriate to view hyperactivity solely in terms of an arousal model. One should keep in mind that the studies of the psychophysiological response pattern in hyperactive children have classified the study population on the basis of a pattern of hyperactive behavior without taking into account the possibility of differential etiology. Thus, hyperactivity related to such conditions as anxiety, phobic reactions, depression, dysphoria, and failure in coping mechanisms could well represent a group in which the hyperactivity was related to a normal or increased arousal level.

In addition to methodological problems relating to the criteria for composing the hyperactive groups, there are also problems in the recording procedures. In reviewing Barkley and Jackson's (1977) discussion of autonomic nervous system activity and stimulant drug effects, one conclusion must be that it is not unexpected that the results are inconsistent. Contradictory findings may well be reflecting methodological shortcomings as much as variations in the populations that have been examined. The measures of state of arousal have been many. In Satterfield's studies, galvanic skin resistance variables were used. In studying Satterfield's and other researchers' reports on electrodermal response pattern in hyperactive children, one is struck by the lack of consistency in terminology as well as procedure. For example, some studies use the term "skin conductance level" (SCL) when galvanic skin response measures actually have been obtained. By simple arithmetic computation, these galvanic skin response data have been converted to SC data. It is not clear that such a conversion is meaningful physiologically. In spite of these differences in terminology, Satterfield and his co-workers have added to our knowledge by suggesting that stimulant drugs must have an effect on central activating mechanisms.

THE PRESENT STUDY

Three groups of children were studied:

1. Children in whom experienced clinicians agreed on the hyperkinesis diagnosis from a behavioral point of view.
2. Children who were referred for hyperactive behavior, but in whom a differential diagnostic evaluation led to a diagnostic classification of "hyperreactivity."
3. Control children with no history of deviant behavior.

The idea was to identify those patients who were referred for hyperactive behavior and in whom the hyperactivity could be related to psychological mechanisms such as anxiety, depression, and coping failure. Thus, the three categories composing the hyperreactive group were:

1. Neurotic reactions associated with anxiety and phobic reactions.
2. Depressive reactions.
3. Coping failure, exemplified by children who are subjected to the expectation of high academic achievement without the necessary intellectual resources to meet these expectations.

Patients with hyperactive behavior associated with autistic traits, mental retardation, or the use of drugs were not included in the study.

More important than excluding certain behavior and personality traits is focusing on what we consider the cardinal symptoms of hyperactivity:

1. Motor hyperactivity
2. Poor impulse control
3. Low frustration tolerance
4. Short attention span
5. Distractibility
6. Aggressiveness
7. Diminished sensitivity to reinforcement

According to Klein and Gittelman-Klein (1971), the hyperkinetic syndrome is characterized by the relatively high intercorrelation between the different symptoms of which the syndrome is composed, and each symptom in itself is neither sufficient nor necessary for establishing the diagnosis. The symptoms of which the syndrome consists will vary from author to author, but in the literature there is nevertheless a considerable amount of agreement between clinicians with regard to what constitutes the central symptoms of the hyperkinetic syndrome. Most of the symptoms mentioned above should be present in order to arrive at the diagnosis, but if these symptoms were present in association with evidence of depression, coping failure, phobic or anxiety reaction, or suspicion of drug-induced behavior problems, the patients were not included in the hyperactive group. In this way, we were able to identify 62 children who satisfied our clinical criteria for hyperactivity.

Procedure

All children who were referred for a hyperactive behavior disorder were evaluated neurologically and neuropsychologically, and complete developmental and anamnestic information was obtained. In addition, SCLs were recorded. A Beckman Dynograph (Type SR) with a Beckman SCL coupler (Type 9844) was used. The electrodes were Beckman's bipotential electrodes with a surface of approximately 64 mm². The electrode paste used was Siemens Elema mingograf electrode cream. Great care was taken to avoid having the electrode paste cover an area larger than the size of the electrode surface. Leakage of electrode paste around the electrode was avoided. The electrodes were attached to the left hand, with the active electrode on the thenar side of the hand and the passive electrode directly opposite on the dorsal side. After the basic SCL was established for a period of 10 minutes, the patient was subjected to 15 presentations of a 1000-Hz, 95-dB tone of 2 seconds duration with interstimulus intervals of 20 seconds.

The SCL parameters evaluated were:

1. Basic SCL.
2. Number of spontaneously occurring changes in the recording during a 120 second period.
3. Number of SCL responses to the auditory stimulation before the responses habituated.

This procedure was common for all three groups—the hyperactive group, the hyperreactive group, and the control group. In addition, the recording was repeated after 60 minutes for the control group and the hyperactive group, but the hyperactive group was given 10 mg of Ritalin immediately after the first recording. The hyperreactive group, also called the "other behavioral pathology" group, was recorded only once.

Results

The results of this study are presented in Table 1. They can be summarized as follows:

1. There is a striking difference in basal SCL between the first session for the control group and the "no-medication" session for the hyperactive group.
2. This difference was greatly reduced 1 hour after 10 mg of Ritalin was administered to the hyperactive group.
3. The "other behavioral pathology" group had a basal SCL that was higher than for any of the other groups.
4. There was no substantial difference between the first and second sessions for the controls. The "no-medication" session for the hyperactive group showed a very low spontaneous activity level, which was significantly increased in the direction of normality 1 hour after 10 mg of Ritalin. The "other behavior pathology" group gave results on this variable that were comparable to the control group.

Table 1.   Summary of skin conductance measures in three behavioral groups studied

	Basal SC level (micromohs)	Spontaneous SC activity during 120 sec	Habituation to 15 1000-Hz 95-dB tones
Controls (N = 10)			
Session I	13.80 SD 9.90[a]	10.30 SD 7.83[a]	13.5 SD 4.74[a]
Session II	15.20 SD 7.80	13.30 SD 4.10	13.5 SD 4.40
Hyperactive (N = 62)			
No medication	5.06 SD 3.63[b]	2.75 SD 3.16[b]	8.47 SD 5.77[a]
10 mg Ritalin	11.24 SD 5.91	6.61 SD 4.11	8.65 SD 5.86
Other behavioral pathology (N = 12)	17.08 SD 6.00	12.39 SD 5.32	9.00 SD 5.60

[a] Not significant.
[b] $p < 0.001$.

5.   With regard to habituation, there was a clear difference between the control group and the two other groups, but the Ritalin did not seem to have any effect on the habituation to the auditory stimulation.

These results are presented graphically in Figure 1.

In Figures 2 and 3, sample recordings from one patient, a hyperactive child, are presented. In each figure, the upper recording is before Ritalin is administered and the lower recording is 1 hour after 10 mg of Ritalin. In Figure 2, the vertical lines indicate the 120-second period during which the spontaneous SCL changes were scored. The pre-Ritalin SCL (upper recording) was 1.41 micromohs. In the lower recording, the SCL curve is displayed 1 hour after administration of 10 mg of Ritalin. The base level after Ritalin is 15.3 micromohs, with a great increase in spontaneously occurring changes in the SCL.

In Figure 3, the curves are obtained from the same patient as in Figure 2, but toward the end of the session and during the presentation of the 95-dB, 1000-Hz tone. In the upper recording, before Ritalin, it is evident that clear responses to the auditory stimuli are poor. However, when the same procedure was repeated 1 hour after administration of 10 mg of Ritalin, the responses to the stimuli are clearly evident. The scoring is based on the number of positive changes in the recording at the correct point after each stimulus, and failure to respond was counted only if there were three successive instances of no response.

Retrospective Data   It appears that the hypothesis postulated initially—that hyperactive children are autonomically hyporeactive and

128   Kløve and Hole

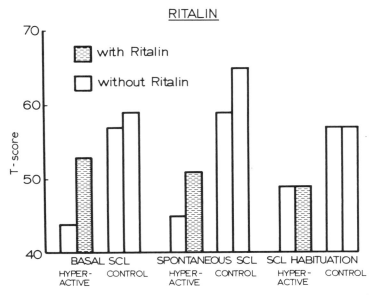

Figure 1.   Graphic presentation of the results on SCL variables with and without Ritalin.

that stimulant drugs act on central activation mechanisms—is supported. The next part of the study concerned possible clues to the etiology of the hyperactive behavior. For this reason, the developmental history and relevant anamnestic information was collected during the intake interviews and then evaluated. The parents or guardians were subjected to an intensive interview with regard to the development of the child and, where indicated, medical and obstetric records were consulted.

Pregnancies in which factors that increase the probability for miscarriage (still-born births, premature delivery, low birth weight, disease, congenital deformaties, mental retardation, or other factors detrimental to normal development) are present are called "risk pregnancies." Some of these factors (for example, use of certain drugs) have a direct causal relationship to the risk itself, and others represent conditions that draw attention to the possibility of a risk. Such risk factors in relationship to pregnancy can be represented by, for example, genetic disposition, the age of the pregnant woman, infections, malnutrition in the mother, roentgen irradiation, or inadequate nutrition of the fetus because of malfunction of the placenta. Children who are considered to be in the so-called high risk category include, according to Nelson, Vaughan, and McKay (1969), those who are "born prematurely, at low or very high

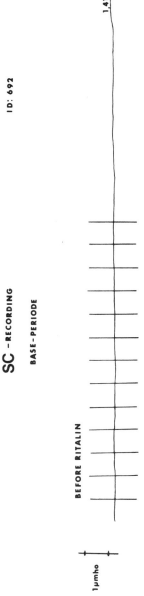
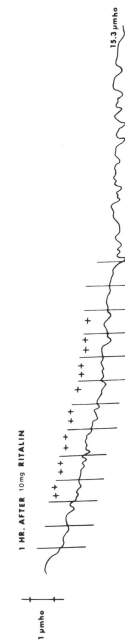

Figure 2.   Sample recording of SCL in a hyperkinetic 6-year-old-boy.

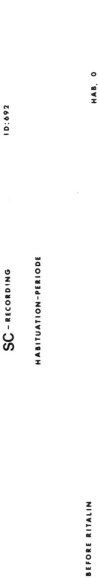

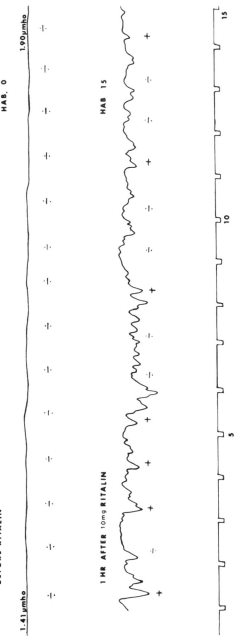

Figure 3.   Sample recording continued. Same patient as in Figure 2.

weight for the gestation age, delivered more than 3 weeks after expected confinement or of multiple pregnancy; delivered operatively or with any unusual obstetric complication; who required resuscitation in the delivery room; born to a mother with infections, any illness during pregnancy, premature rupture of membranes, toxemia, drug addition, and with a history of taking any of the medications listed in the table during pregnancy." With regard to infection, it is especially rubella that has been associated with damage to the fetus. This includes deformities in the cardiovascular system as well as the central nervous system, most commonly occurring if the mother is exposed to an infection of rubella during the first 3 months of pregnancy (Reid, 1959). Many other viral infections are suspected of having less serious consequences for the child. Pasamanick and Knobloch (1966) maintain that there seems to be a relationship between urinary infections in the mother and prematurity of the child.

The area of "risk factor" research is complicated. In the present study, an attempt was made to investigate the extent to which deviations in pregnancy or early development were associated with the definition of hyperactivity that was arrived at in the first part of this paper (hyperactive behavior associated with low autonomic reactivity that normalized after administration of Ritalin).

Only a few of the variables investigated are presented here. In Table 2, the risk factors with the highest incidence are listed. Vaginal bleeding occurring throughout the pregnancy was included in the factors. Precipitous delivery was defined as delivery taking place within 4 hours of onset of labor, and protracted delivery was defined as delivery taking place 20 hours or more after onset of labor. It was difficult to obtain information corresponding to the categories listed in Table 2 from the control population. However, the occurrence of abnormality during pregnancy and the perinatal period in the hyperactive group is clearly deviant.

Table 2.   Risk factors with highest incidence ($N = 62$)

	N	%
Vaginal bleeding	7	11
Precipitous delivery	15	24
Protracted delivery	14	19
Cyanosis at delivery	14	19
Neonatal feeding problem	14	19
Fever above 40°C	7	11
Convulsive episodes	6	11
O_2 at delivery	6	10

Functional Deficits All 62 patients were subjected to an extensive neuropsychological examination. The symptoms listed in Table 3 have been arrived at on the basis of neuropsychological test data and anamnestic information. The entries in the table are self-explanatory. However, the last entry, "head injury," should be explained further. Information about sustained head injury was obtained as an index of accident proneness. Thirty percent of the group had had one or several significant head injuries. It should be emphasized that head injuries in this context were not trivial incidents, but injuries that had one or several of the following consequences:

1. Unconsciousness
2. Skull fracture
3. Craniotomy
4. Generally accepted criteria for commotio cerebri

The high incidence of head injuries supports the general impression that these children are especially accident prone.

Birth Weight In Figure 4, the distribution of birth weight for the patient sample is given. The mean birth weight was 3370 g. By inspecting Figure 4, one can observe an overrepresentation in the low and the high ends of the distribution. Eight of the patients had a birth weight of 2500 g or less, and five of the children had a birth weight of 4500 g or more.

Table 4 shows that 57.5% of the children were born after 40 weeks of pregnancy, and 91.5% were born between 37 and 42 weeks of pregnancy. On the basis of these data, it seems that the occurrence of prematurity is not unusually high. However, by using another method of analysis, an entirely different picture emerges. By evaluating the birth weight in relationship to the gestational age (Bjerkedal, Bakketeig, and Lehmann, 1973), a different distribution occurs.

Table 3.   Table of functional deficits ($N = 62$)

	N	%
Impaired motor function	33	53
Delayed motor development	16	25
Speech impairment	14	23
Delayed language development	23	36
Writing difficulties	20	32
Reading difficulties	20	32
Memory impairment	7	11
Head injury	19	30

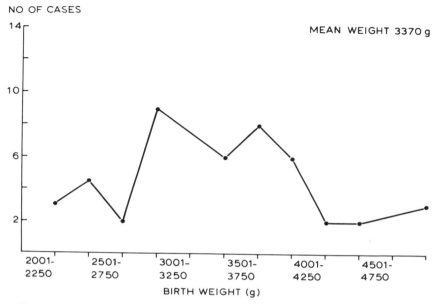

NO OF CASES

MEAN WEIGHT 3370 g

BIRTH WEIGHT (g)

Figure 4. Graphic presentation of birth weight of the hyperkinetic patients ($N = 59$).

Figure 5 shows the percentile distribution for the group based on the material presented by Bjerkedal et al. (1973). The figure shows that the percentile distribution for this group is clearly left-skewed—66.1% of the patients fell at the 50th percentile, 42.4% at the 25th percentile, and 28.8% at the 10th percentile. This means that the incidence of birth weight below what is accepted as the critical limit is almost three times as high as would be expected in a normal population. At the same time, 15.2% of the patients have a birth weight too high for their gestational age (90th percentile). This implies that 44% of this patient group fell within the two extreme areas of a normal distribution (below or above two standard deviations from the mean).

Table 4. Gestational age distribution table ($N = 59$)

	Gestational age (weeks)											
	32	33	34	35	36	37	38	39	40	41	42	43
Number of babies	1	0	0	1	1	6	3	4	34	3	4	2

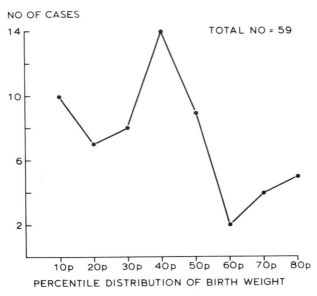

NO OF CASES

TOTAL NO = 59

PERCENTILE DISTRIBUTION OF BIRTH WEIGHT

Figure 5. Graphic presentation of the percentile distribution of the relationship between birth weight and gestational age.

Conclusions

The present study has demonstrated four main points:

1. By careful clinical screening of the hyperactive patient group, it was possible to identify a group of hyperactive patients in whom the psychophysiological findings were interpreted to represent evidence of a state of hypoarousal. Administration of a central nervous system stimulant normalized the hypoaroused state.

2. Children displaying hyperactive behavior in whom psychological mechanisms appear to be a decisive factor in producing the symptoms did not demonstrate the same psychophysiological evidence of hypoarousal.

3. By reviewing the restrospective data for the hypoaroused hyperactive children, it was possible to demonstrate the occurrence of a high incidence of "risk factors" in pregnancy and delivery. By evaluating data obtained on the child's development, a high incidence of deviant developmental patterns was established.

4. The more striking finding was the overrepresentation of dysmature births in the hyperactive group with psychophysiological evidence of hypoarousal.

The practical implications of the results of this study are many. It is felt that careful application of psychophysiological techniques such as SCL registration can yield results that may be of importance in both the clinical and the pharmacological management of the hyperactive child.

In this as in other clinical studies, the nature of the study population imposed limitations on the experimental design. One such limitation is that we did not obtain data on the effect of Ritalin on the normal control group. When seen in relationship to the question of primary interest, it was felt that the problems of obtaining permission to give Ritalin to the control population were too great. However, in our experience, children with normal SCLs react the same way to stimulant drugs as do children with low SCLs—with an increase in autonomic reactivity. In a recent paper, Rapoport et al. (1978) reported that there is no evidence of paradoxical reaction to stimulant drugs in normal as compared with hyperactive children; the changes occur with the baseline at a different point on the arousal continuum. This is a conclusion that our own clinical experience supports.

One advantage of using a measure of autonomic reactivity is that the differential diagnostic decisions are easier to make. The psychophysiological variables also give guidance with regard to evaluating the patient's reaction to the drug and establishing to what extent the patient is a responder. As indicated above, we feel that a number of hyperactive children can be classified as hyperreactive, i.e., the hyperactive behavior can be adequately explained in purely psychological terms and consequently should be treated with psychological methods. The problem is, in our experience, that some of the hyperreactive children show attenuation of the symptoms when placed on stimulant drugs. We feel, however, that central stimulants should be reserved for those patients in whom a deficit in central activating mechanism can be demonstrated and who have responded with normalization of the psychophysiological variables with a trial-dose of a central stimulant. It should also be emphasized that treatment with stimulant drugs should be accompanied by appropriate medical, psychological, and educational treatment and that drug treatment should be viewed as only one element in the comprehensive care of these patients.

In summary, this study has confirmed our two hypotheses. A group of hyperactive children can be identified in whom it is possible to demonstrate a state of hypoarousal. In these children there seems to be a convincing accumulation of deviation in pregnancy and perinatal events as well as in a number of functional parameters. The association between hypoarousal and accumulation of a large number of so-called risk factors and functional deficits raises the very complicated question of the etiology of hyperkinetic behavior associated with hypoarousal. Clearly, the possibility of identifying two main groups of hyperactives exists, one in whom hyperactive behavior has primarily a psychological etiology and another in whom it has primarily a neurogenic etiology.

REFERENCES

Barkley, R. A. 1977. A review of stimulant drug research with hyperactive children. J. Child Psychol. Psychiatry 18:137–165.

Barkley, R. A., and Jackson, T. L., Jr. 1977. Hyperkinesis, autonomic nervous system activity and stimulant drug effects. J. Child Psychol. Psychiatry 18:347–357.

Bjerkedal, T., Bakketeig, L., and Lehmann, E. H. 1973. Percentile of birth weight of single, live births at different gestation periods. Acta Paediatr. Scand. 62:449–457.

Boydstun, J. A., Ackerman, P. T., Stevens, D. A., Clemens, S. D., Peters, J. E., and Dykman, R. A. 1968. Physiologic and motor conditioning and generalization in children with minimal brain dysfunction. Conditional Reflex 3:81–104.

Bradley, C. 1937. The behavior of children receiving benzedrine. Am. J. Psychiatry 94:577–585.

Duffy, E. 1962. Activation and Behavior. John Wiley & Sons, Inc., New York.

Eysenck, H. J. 1970. The Biological Basis of Personality. Charles C Thomas, Springfield, Ill.

Klein, D. F., and Gittelman-Klein, R. 1971. Diagnosis of minimal brain dysfunction and hyperkinetic syndrome. In C. K. Conners (ed.), Clinical Use of Stimulant Drugs in Children. American Elsevier Publishing Co., New York.

Luria, A. 1973. The Working Brain: An Introduction to Neuropsychology. Penguin, London.

Malmo, R. B. 1959. Activation: A neuropsychological dimension. Psychol. Rev. 66:367–386.

Moruzzi, G., and Magoun, H. W. 1949. Brain stem reticular formation and activation of the EEG. Clin. Neurophysiol. 1:455–473.

Nelson, W. E., Vaughan, V. C., and McKay, R. J. (eds.) 1969. Textbook of Pediatrics. W. B. Saunders Co., London.

Pasamanick, B., and Knobloch, H. 1966. Retrospective studies on the epidemiology of reproductive causality: Old and new. Merrill-Palmer Q. 12:7–26.

Rapoport, J. L., Bucksbaum, M. S., Zahn, P., Wiengartner, H., Ludlaw, C., and Mikkelsen, F. J. 1978. Dextroamphetamine: Cognitive and behavioral effects in normal prepubertal boys. Science 199:560–563.

Reid, D. E. 1959. Remote effects of obstetrical hazards on the development of the child. A review of the problem. J. Obstet. Gynaecol. Br. Empire 66:709–720.

Satterfield, J. H., and Dawson, M. E. 1971. Electrodermal correlates of hyperactivity in children. Psychophysiology 8:191–198.

Satterfield, J. H., Atoian, G., Brashears, A. C., Burleigh, A. C., and Dawson, M. E. 1974. Electrodermal studies in minimal brain dysfunction children. In C. K. Conners (ed.), Clinical Use of Stimulant Drugs in Children. American Elsevier Publishing Co., New York.

Discussion of
"The Hyperkinetic Syndrome"

Virginia I. Douglas

The question of using psychophysiological measures in the study of hyperactive children is one over which I have a great deal of concern. In attempting to determine the usefulness of this approach, I have continually met with inconclusive results. Dr. Kløve has suggested some of the basic reasons why this is a common problem, such as the overwhelming number of measures of arousal. Unfortunately, there are many cases of pseudosophistication in this area, since appropriate measures or means of taking such measures have not been agreed on.

For example, we have found differences between hyperactives and normals in physiological measures if the measures are taken at a time when the children are attending to a task. The hyperactives have appeared to be at a lower level of arousal than the normals.

However, the general concept of "level of arousal" has not really proved to be too useful to us. I believe that the ability of the child to adapt his level of arousal to the needs of the situation will perhaps be a more important construct to study. Perhaps the term attention is more appropriate than general arousal level.

A major difference between Dr. Kløve's study and the work I have been involved with is the very different subject sample. We deliberately screen out all children with histories suggestive of brain injury.

Methodologically, there is one point I would like to mention. Dr. Kløve collected data on all the hyperactive children, first off drugs and then in the drug condition. We have consistently found that hyperactives behave differently during a retest situation. If it is a simple task, the performance usually deteriorates. It would have been interesting had Dr. Kløve used a cross-over design to clear up that point.

Theoretically, it is interesting to speculate on treatment implications if hyperactive children are indeed at a lower arousal level. I would like to see psychophysiological studies accompanied by behavioral data where one could see how children perform on various tasks when arousal levels are manipulated. If we could combine the behavioral and physiological measures, I think we would be in business.

Response to Discussion

Hallgrim Kløve

I would like to comment on a few points in Dr. Virginia Douglas' discussion of my paper. I do not see that it is much of an argument that other papers have given inconclusive results in regard to psychophysiological variables in hyperactive children. This argument is only appropriate to the extent that these other papers have used similar psychophysiological recording techniques and have employed the same criteria for selecting the patients. I am not aware of any other study that has used skin conductance level under the same conditions we have employed and used patient groups that have been selected with consideration of the same differential diagnostic factors. Another point is that several studies claim that they have used skin conductance levels when in fact skin resistance levels have been recorded and converted to skin conductance level equivalents by simple arithmetic. This may be one of the most important objections to these studies. Analyzing both our own data and other studies, there can be little doubt that skin resistance is a much more unstable physiological variable than skin conductance. Nevertheless, I am pleased to see that one of Dr. Douglas' doctoral students has concluded that there seems to be a trend in the literature suggesting that hyperactive children are underaroused and that an increased arousal level is a prerequisite for improved behavior. I think we are going to see additional studies with results in this direction because improvement in psychophysiological techniques will increase the stability of the physiological measures.

However, it is important to define carefully the criteria for including a child in a hyperactive group, since the results are naturally going to be influenced by the characteristics of patients one includes in the study. This brings me to another point in Dr. Douglas' remarks—that she felt that our children represented a very different sample than the children she works with. I think I understood Dr. Douglas to say that she in her studies explicitly excluded children with a history that would imply neurological dysfunction or damage. In our study we did not do this. The initial criteria for including or excluding a child were strictly a clinical and a behavioral evaluation. I think it is important to repeat a couple of conclusions from our study to clear up this difference in Dr. Douglas' patients and my patients. In those of our children who had low autonomic reactivity and in whom the autonomic reactivity normalized after administration of Ritalin, we found an overwhelming accumulation of developmental risk factors, and evidence of neurological damage and dysfunction. One of the more striking findings was that the group was heavily overrepresented by children who were "small-for-date babies." Thus we did not prescreen our children for presence or absence of evidence of neurological dysfunction or damage; the starting point was that they presented with hyperactive behavior. In this regard there is no question that Dr. Douglas and I talk about different patient groups. In our patient population, with normal autonomic reactivity but hyperactive behavior, we were in general not able to demonstrate evidence of neurological dysfunction or damage or deviant developmental history.

Finally, I agree with Dr. Douglas with regard to the concept of arousal. In the beginning of my talk I briefly discussed the arousal concept. The arousal concept has been widely used both in the psychological and neurophysiological literature, and as a theoretical construct I think it is both helpful and useful, but it would be difficult to agree on a psychological and/or neurophysiological definition of arousal that would clarify the complex interaction between psychological and neurophysiological processes.

Method and Theory for Psychopharmacology with Children

C. Keith Conners
and
Karen C. Wells

There are two reasons why drugs are used with children: the first is that they are sometimes effective in treating symptoms that interfere with the child's adaptive functioning, and the second is that drugs may offer insights into the etiology and pathophysiology underlying the disturbances of overt behavior. There are, in other words, therapeutic and theoretical, or practical and scientific, bases for the use of psychopharmacologic agents. It is taken for granted by most clinicians in the field that the use of drugs can be justified on purely pragmatic grounds, regardless of whether or not a particular scientific rationale for their effects is available. This is, of course, a common stance in therapeutics generally, where we have become familiar with many treatments that are applied well in advance of explanations as to how and why they work. It is a rare exception in children's psychopharmacology to find studies that are carried out for purely theoretical reasons, such as Rapoport et al.'s (1978) recent study of stimulant effects in normal children. It seems quite likely that future studies will become even more restricted to investigations within a clinical treatment context, and even more constrained by the ethical and cultural antipathy to pure experimentation with children.

Yet it also seems obvious that there are rapidly diminishing returns in studies that merely ask which drug removes which symptom, or which drug is more effective. Such questions are useful in the early stages of

---

The authors gratefully acknowledge the assistance of Lois G. Imber, who assisted in the data collection.

141

psychopharmacology, when drugs have not been tested at all, or when new drugs must be compared with old ones for safety and efficacy. In the past two decades the "safety and efficacy" criteria have dominated most of the research. Despite this necessary empirical approach, it is not uncommon to find that practitioners are dissatisfied with the state of knowledge. Although it may be reassuring to them to learn that we have carefully compared drugs X, Y, and Z in double-blind controlled trials with populations A, B, or C, this information is seldom translatable into guidelines for clinical application in particular cases.

Moreover, recent reviews have repeatedly argued that treating children on the basis of symptoms alone leads to excessive and irrational use of drugs and a tendency to ignore the social and nonbiological contributions to the illness. In our judgment, future childhood psychopharmacology will permit treatment only when there is clear theoretical understanding of the contributions of neurobiologic factors to symptom formation. There is, of course, no reason that purely socially caused disturbances cannot and should not be treated with pharmacologic agents, but it is a strong and widely held belief that behaviorally caused disturbances require behavioral interventions, and biologically caused disturbances may allow one to use biologic interventions. Whether logically and scientifically defensible or not, such an attitude has had a strong impact on our ability to study drugs with children, and will have more and more restrictive effects in the future. It therefore seems incumbent that the psychopharmacology of the future for young children must address itself to theoretical explanations based on the way biological and environmental variables relate to maladaptive functioning in addition to more pragmatic goals; and it must begin to specify in detail methods for deciding what children in what context should receive what treatments in what combinations.

In this paper we would like to outline a theory of how one class of drugs—stimulants—acts to produce changes in one class of childhood behavior disturbance—the hyperkinetic reaction of childhood. We will illustrate some of the applications of this theory by two case studies that employ single-subject experimental methodology, and then attempt to draw some general implications for future investigations. Our interest in this paper is the general one of addressing the methods, assumptions, and principles by which we think progress in the field will be made rather than in a detailed statement of the theory or its empirical tests.

We proposed in 1963 (Conners and Eisenberg, 1963) that stimulant effects in hyperkinetics could be accounted for by two actions: an increase in alertness or arousal, and an increase in inhibition. Inhibition is conceived as a property of the developing nervous system that prevents immediate motor discharge in response to internal or external stimulation. Arousal is the phasic or tonic property of the nervous system that regulates excitability of particular cortical processors. Arousal affects performance according to the familiar inverted U-shaped function, with low arousal and high arousal states both leading to disruption of task performance, especially sustained attention.

We consider the primary symptoms of hyperkinesis to be of two kinds: disinhibition of motor behavior—commonly referred to as restlessness, fidgetiness, impulsivity, and distractibility—and symptoms due to either excessive or inadequate arousal, leading to the other core symptoms of lack of sustained attention and certain learning disabilities. Although the two processes are conceived as orthogonol to each other, they clearly interact; a certain degree of alertness is required for inhibitory mechanisms to come into play and vice versa. However, one process may be affected by external insults and the other not; one may be held constant while the other varies, so that some children will have symptoms of impulsivity without inattentiveness, and vice versa.

More importantly, both processes may be independently influenced by environmental structure. Although we have spoken of these two processes primarily from the reference point of the nervous system (as constructs inferred from behavior in certain stimulus situations), it is fundamental to recognize that both processes are also environmentally influenced. Environmental contingencies and structure will limit the expression of motor behavior and bring it under control; indeed, throughout the course of ontongenetic development internal structures depend for their organization on external structures, as Piaget has clearly shown us. We also know that novelty, complexity, contrast, and other environmental properties influence arousal and orientation to the external world, as Sokolov (1963), for example, has demonstrated so clearly. In this two-factor model of symptom formation we can think of different symptoms coming into play, depending on the shifting balance between arousal and inhibition, and we can also think of their expression as dependent on the shifting features of the external environment. A strongly disinhibited nervous system will lead to impulsive behavior across a wide range of values of arousal and a wide range of degrees of environmental structure and control. A minimally disinhibited nervous system may still lead to impulsivity under an environment with little external structure. A very underaroused child may still function adequately in a highly novel stimulus environment. A number of interesting predictions can be made from this model, but we simply wish to emphasize here that drug effects will be understood only if we remember to take into account degree of external constraint (inhibition) and degree of external excitation (arousal). Different drug effects in home and school, or between two kinds of classroom or two kinds of homes, need to be analyzed for these two sets of orthogonal environmental properties, as well as for their biological counterparts in the nervous system.

We believe that stimulant drugs have the property of increasing the phasic arousal potential of the nervous system, probably through direct actions on the ascending reticular activating system, and that these drugs also probably have effects on frontal lobe structures that mediate voluntary motor inhibition and reflective behavior. However, these effects will depend on the extent to which arousing and inhibiting factors in the child's environment are present. Recent behavioral studies of the hyperkinetic child show quite clearly that external constraints in the form of reward contingencies can greatly modify the expression of symptoms relating to on-task behavior and out-of-seat behavior. These contingencies control normal child behavior as well, but either the magnitude or schedule of the reinforcements may need to be adjusted for a child whose nervous system has suffered perinatal insults or genetic handicap or developmental delay.

Let us now turn to some illustrations of pharmacological-environmental interactive effects from our recent work in a children's inpatient unit—a setting where both the methods of observation and the control over the environment afford good conditions for studying the mutual interactions we have discussed.*

Our first case, Billy, is a 9-year-old black male whose referral problems included slow academic development in all areas, very short attention span, poor concentration, unmanageable behavior in class, and aggression toward peers, adults, and objects. Physical examination showed a boy with peculiar facies, including protruding jaw and upper teeth, small ears, and slightly exotropic eyes. Neurologic exam showed poor right-left and two-point discrimination, poor persistence, poor tandem gait, and figure copying. EEG was considered abnormal because of excessive fast and sharp activity, but with no seizure foci. WISC IQs were Full Scale 80, with a 78 Verbal and 85 Performance.

A variant of a single case withdrawal design was used to evaluate the effects of Dexedrine, Ritalin, and self-control procedures. Three behaviors whose modification was considered crucial to academic per-

---

* These two studies were designed and carried out by Karen Wells with the assistance of Lois Imber and Alan Delamater.

formance were targeted in the classroom. During all phases a trained observer was in the classroom and recorded gross motor behavior (excessive movement in or out of seat, such as squirming, rocking, standing, or jumping in seat or walking or running around the room); inappropriate noise and vocalizations (singing, humming, whistling, yelling, talking without permission, pencil tapping, clapping, slamming desks or books); and off-task behavior (looking away from his assigned task for more than 5 seconds of each 20-second recording interval). The occurrence or nonoccurrence of each of these behaviors was scored in consecutive 20-second intervals. On 29% of the observation days a second trained reliability observer was stationed in the classroom and recorded the same behaviors. Reliability between the two observers for occurrence only (a stringent criterion) was 0.78 for gross motor, 0.75 for noise and vocalizations, and 0.86 for off-task behavior. Deviant peer interactions and gross motor behaviors were also monitored out of the classroom in an unstructured play situation using direct interval sampling and scales from the Children's Behavior Inventory (CBI) of Burdock and Hardesty (1967).

Results are presented in Figures 1 and 2. Off-task behavior occurred in about 50% of the recording intervals during the initial baseline phase. The introduction of Dexedrine in Phase 2 resulted in deterioration of this behavior to about 60%. In session 24, Ritalin was introduced and results show improvement over baseline phases in off-task behavior, which occurred at about 23% during this phase.

Having determined that Billy appeared to be a Ritalin responder, we were then interested in any additional improvement that might be obtained using a self-control program. In Phase 5 a self-control program was introduced. A tape recorder with randomly spaced "beeps" was placed on Billy's desk along with two bowls, one empty and one containing red poker chips. During the first three days (sessions 33 through 35), an experimenter sat by Billy, placed a red chip into the empty bowl whenever a beep occurred and Billy was on task. During sessions 36 through 38, Billy monitored his own behavior by placing chips in his bowl if he was on task when the "beep" occurred. The experimenter sat nearby and merely observed. Beginning in session 39, the experimenter was no longer present in the classroom. Billy was given the recorder, bowls, and chips and told to cash in his self-administered chips after class. Earned chips were exchangeable for tangible and edible treats during the afternoon snack period. In Phase 6, the self-control program continued while Ritalin was withdrawn and replaced by a placebo. In the last phase, Ritalin was again administered along with the self-control program. Off-task behavior decreased to essentially zero levels in Phase

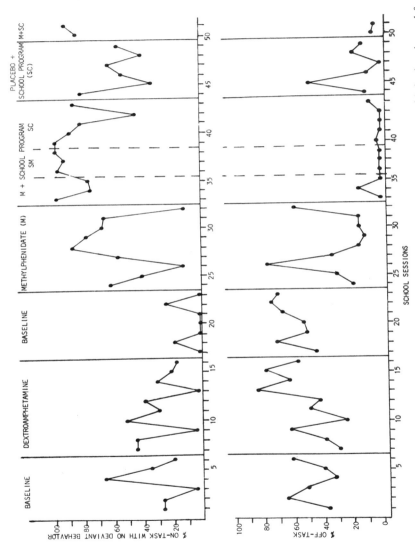

Figure 1. Patient Billy's on-task behavior. Each data point represents approximately 40 to 60 samples of behavior observed for 20-second periods during ½ hour of class time. Data show increased on-task with methylphenidate (M), and even better performance when self-monitoring (SM) and self-control (SC) procedures are introduced. Removing the drug leads to some loss of control, which is reinstated when the drug is reintroduced in the final phase.

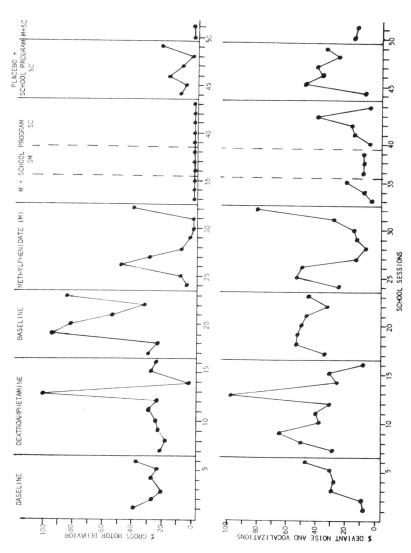

Figure 2. Patient Billy's gross motor and deviant vocalizations. Neither behavior was specifically reinforced by the self-control program, but gross motor behavior is strongly affected by the self-control procedure, and deviant vocalizations are better under the combination of drug and self-control than with either treatment alone.

5. When Ritalin was withdrawn, off-task behavior increased only slightly to around 20%. When Ritalin was again reinstated, the effect in Phase 5 was replicated.

Figure 2 presents similar results for gross motor behavior. Ritalin alone was not as effective as Ritalin plus self-control, as can be seen in Phase 5 when gross motor behavior dropped to zero. This represents an important side effect of the self-control program, since gross motor behavior was not explicitly reinforced. When Ritalin was withdrawn, gross motor behavior increased slightly to about 10%. In the final phase Ritalin and self-control combined again resulted in 0 percent gross motor behavior.

Inappropriate noise and vocalizations show a slightly different course. Neither Dexedrine, Ritalin, nor self-control result in substantial improvement alone. However, the combination of Ritalin plus the self-control program (Phases 5 and 7) results in decreases to around 15%.

In contrast to these results in the classroom setting, which in addition to being highly structured had further structure in the form of self-

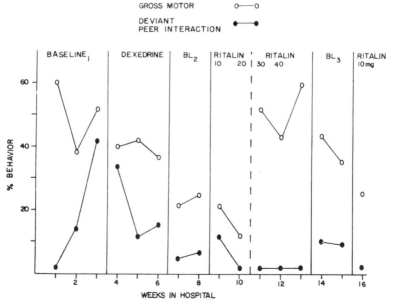

Figure 3.   Patient Billy's direct observation of gross motor and deviant peer behavior on the hospital ward. In contrast to the classroom, these behaviors are not affected by the treatment program. Each data point represents approximately 30 minutes of interval sampling observation.

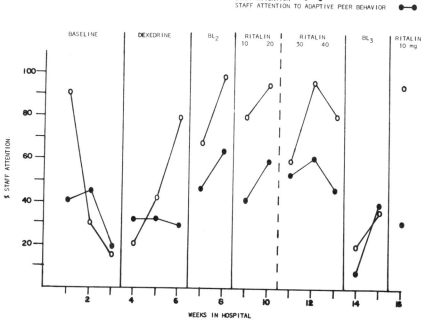

Figure 4.   Staff attention for patient Billy. Each time a child was scored for adaptive peer behavior any staff response occurring within 10 seconds was scored. Note the increased staff attention once drug therapy was begun. Staff attention is significantly correlated with the deviant peer behavior shown in the previous figure.

monitoring and self-control programs superimposed, results obtained on the ward in a free play situation were quite different. Figure 3 shows the direct interval sampling measures of gross motor and deviant peer interactions obtained on the ward. Although equally reliable, these data show no relationship between drug manipulations and overt behavior. Instead, as may be seen in Figure 4, direct observations of staff attention and staff attention to adaptive peer behavior reveals that staff behavior is correlated with the changes in the child's behavior. This has been one of our most striking findings—in the unstructured ward environment the behavior of the children is largely under the control of staff attention. The rank order correlation between amount of staff attention and gross motor activity, for example, is −0.59. Clearly the drug effect is either being overridden by a more powerful set of environmental contingencies or shows itself in performance only under conditions where a certain degree of structure either additively or interactively works with the drug to control external behavior. Within the classroom setting itself, it would appear that manipulating the degree of task structure by the self-control procedure further enhances the drug effect. Figure 5 shows that neither a visual-motor task nor staff nurse ratings on the CBI reveal any drug effect in this case.

One related finding of interest is the concurrent physiological recording of peripheral vasoconstriction and electromyographic activity during the drug phases. Figure 6 shows that, although Dexedrine does not produce vasoconstriction, Ritalin does, and Dexedrine does not affect frontalis electromyographic activity, whereas Ritalin does. We have found these same results in several other cases in which the amount of

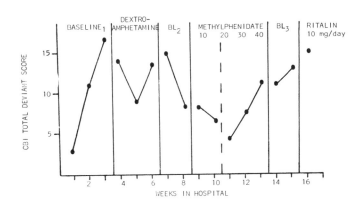

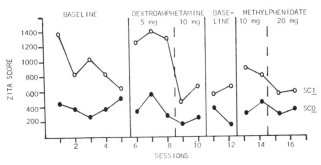

Figure 5.   Lack of drug effects on nurses' observations of deviant behavior (Children's Behavior Inventory) and a visual-motor tracking task (ZITA). Note similarity of deviant behavior during initial baseline to deviant peer observations of Figure 3, which suggests that staff attention (shown in Figure 4) accounts for these "honeymoon" effects.

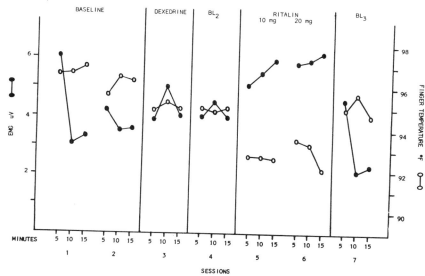

Figure 6.   Electromyogram recorded from frontalis muscle and digital temperature show response to Ritalin but not Dexedrine.

these effects is also related to clinical effects, suggesting that increased muscle tension and peripheral vasoconstriction may be indicative of central adrenergic effects correlated with clinical improvement. We intend to pursue these findings in further studies.

Our second case illustration is Tommy, a 7-year-old white male who was referred for treatment of excessive activity level, limited academic achievement, verbal and physical aggression to classmates and siblings, lying, stealing, and self-injurious behavior such as repeatedly reopening wounds. Interestingly, referral was made following Tommy's unfortunate transfer to an unstructured classroom when he was found attempting to jump from a second-story window. Neurologic examination revealed difficulty with figure tracing, tandem gait forward and backward, poor persistence, and poor right-left discrimination on self and observer. Physical anomalies included thick facies and epicanthal folds covering the tear ducts. He was functioning at a kindergarten level in all academic performance areas. On the WISC-R, Tommy received a Verbal IQ of 98 and a Performance IQ of 77. Auditory skills, including discrimination, memory, and integration, were all very poor. Social history revealed a very erratic and disruptive family situation, including marital conflict and divorce, removal from the maternal home, and harsh discipline by the father.

An A, B, BC, C single case design was used to assess the effects of stimulants and a self-control program on Tommy's classroom behavior. Reliability between the two observers was obtained on 36% of the observation days. For gross motor behavior, reliability was 0.74, for off-task behavior, 0.84, for noise and vocalizations, 0.92, and for on-task with no deviant behavior reliability, 0.95.

Figure 7 shows that, during baseline phase, off-task behavior averaged 90%, gross motor averaged 35%, and inappropriate noise and vocalizations averaged 25%. When Ritalin was introduced all school behaviors improved. However, Tommy experienced a marked behavioral deterioration on the ward and it was decided to discontinue Ritalin and begin Dexedrine. Off-task behavior decreased to an average of 33% while gross motor behavior gradually decelerated across the phase, averaging 24% (Figure 8).

Noise and vocalizations decreased for most of the phase to 14%. The greatest improvements for Tommy, as for Billy, resulted from the com-

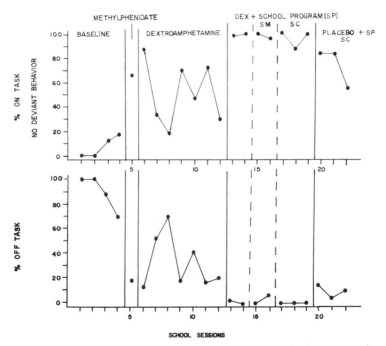

Figure 7.   Patient Tommy's on-task behavior. Methylphenidate improves classroom behavior, but is withdrawn because of disruptive effects on ward behavior. Dexedrine plus self-monitoring and self-control produce maximal improvement in the classroom.

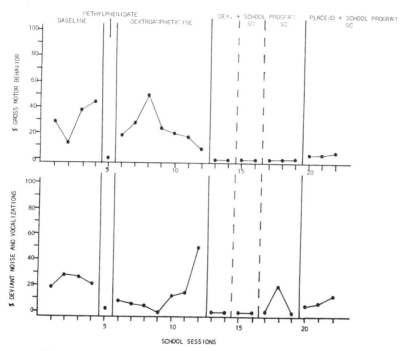

Figure 8.   Gross motor and deviant vocalizations for patient Tommy.

bination of medication and self-control procedures. All behaviors decreased to essentially zero levels when both treatments were combined. Finally, in the last phase, when Dexedrine was withdrawn and the school program alone was in effect, all three behaviors were essentially maintained at low levels.

We have presented these two cases to illustrate both the application of single case methodology using highly reliable direct observations to the study of drug effects and the interaction between drug effects and environmental structure in the form of self-control procedures and variations from classroom to nonclassroom settings. Whether one conceptualizes the findings in terms of summative or interactive environmental and drug effects, the lesson seems clear: drug effects cannot be understood apart from a careful analysis of the context in which they occur. We have chosen to emphasize the concept of "structure" as the total set of external constraints operating to control and limit behavior, either in the form of formal ecologic variables such as the number of persons in the immediate environment or the set of reinforcement contingencies operating to control behavior.

This type of variable can be manipulated with a particular task, such as the visual-motor tracking task called the ZITA (Zero Input Tracking Analyzer). The child is required to track a moving target, producing an output of zero crossings whose integrated value gives an error score. In the simple task (I) the child traces the moving light with simple analog control-stick movements. In the complex (Isc) task he must simultaneously monitor and respond to other lights requiring a left or right button push, thus placing a dual-processing demand on performance.

Figure 9 illustrates the differential impairment effect of a tranquilizing drug on these two types of demand. In Figure 9 we see that deterioration of performance due to Haldol is more apparent on the more complex task. In Figure 10, we see how stimulants act to improve the more complex task. In general, the more complex or demanding task is more

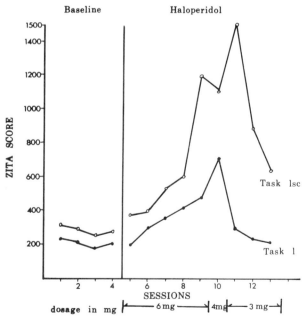

Figure 9.   Zero Input Tracking Analyzer (ZITA) test results. Task I requires simple manual tracking of moving light, while Task Isc requires tracking plus responding to intermittent lights with the other hand. Impairment due to haloperidol more marked under more complex task demands. Patient was a 12-year-old suicidal schizophrenic boy.

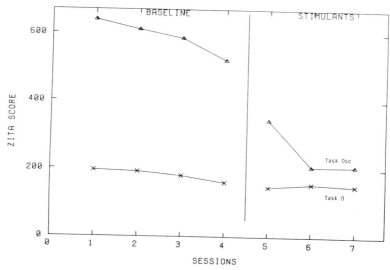

Figure 10. Improvement of ZITA performance with stimulants. Data represents mean performance for four subjects. Task O is simple analog tracking, and task Osc requires monitoring and responding to lights with the other hand.

"drug sensitive," but what this really means is that the range of task demands will determine both whether or not the child's dysfunction is apparent and whether the drug will have any perceived effect.

If our two-factor theory is correct, then for each child there will be some range of structure or limit on the expression of impulsive behavior that is optimal for his performance; and there will be some range or limit of novelty, complexity, or physiological arousal that is optimal for performance. These values should be different for hyperkinetics and normals. Indeed, this might be the most powerful way to operationalize what we mean by calling a child hyperkinetic—the values of the parameters of environmental inhibitors and arousers that lead to optimal performance. Stimulants may be expected to shift those values toward those of the normal child.

Consider for example, Kagan's Matching Familiar Figures Test (MFFT), which requires the child to match a standard figure to one of several slightly discriminable alternatives. The child can do this quickly and make a lot of errors (and be called impulsive), or slowly with few errors (and be called reflective). Normal values for this test will be a function of the particular difficulty of the discriminations required, the number of response alternatives, and implicit payoff contingencies (i.e., if the child were to be punished for errors of commission he would become more reflective, whereas if he were punished for time delays he would become more impulsive). What distinguishes the normal child from a hyperactive child in this task is that the hyperactive child spontaneously makes more impulsive errors for the particular values of the restraining parameters that the test employs. However, we could easily bring his performance into the normal range by either punishing impulsivity or rewarding reflectivity. The amount of punishment or reward would then be an index of how deviant the child is from the normal child. When we treat such a child with drugs and "normalize" his behavior, we are in effect saying that the amount of the parameters then required to produce reflective behavior are the same as for the normal child. What we are suggesting is that by varying these parameters we can determine the extent to which the child deviates from normal as well as measure the conditions under which the drugs alter behavior.

One implication of this analysis is that even the normal child has some set of parameters on a given task that regulates his impulsive behavior, and these might also be altered by drugs, inasmuch as drugs alter effects of punishment or reward and hence the payoff matrix governing the particular task. Similarly, if we hold such parameters constant and vary the interest, novelty, or complexity of the task, we can expect that there will be some optimal level of arousal for the normal child that will regulate performance levels; if the hyperactive child is underarousable, he may require more novelty or complexity or interest to attain the same performance levels as the normal child.

In summary, we see the following developments taking place in future psychopharmacology for the hyperkinetic child. We will see a development of assessment situations at home and school and in the child's natural social environment in which two major variables will be systematically varied: the amount of restraining, inhibitory forces required to limit impulsive discharge of motor behavior, and the amount of stimulus complexity, novelty, and the like required to energize or activate behavior to optimal levels. Such an assessment will operationally define degree of deviance along the dimensions of inhibition and excitation, and will serve to measure the effects of drugs in normalizing behavior along these two dimensions. We will come to learn what combination of environmental modifications along these dimensions produce optimal performance, and where drugs will need to be introduced to add to or multiply the effects of environmental manipulations.

Our two case studies clearly show that behavior modification techniques in combination with stimulant medication provide the most effective treatment approach for some individuals. Even though medication alone and self-control alone apparently resulted in reductions in maladaptive school behaviors from baseline when phase averages are compared, it is clear that the two approaches combined result in the greatest improvement. These results appear discrepant from those of Gittelman-Klein et al.'s recent group study (personal communication) in which behavioral approaches were demonstrated to add insignificantly to drug therapy. However, these two studies illustrate an important point of concern to the practicing clinician: group studies that generate statistically significant effects from average group data are invaluable aids in narrowing the range of effective treatment alternatives. However, individuals within a group in one of these studies may vary greatly in response to this same treatment. Thus, group studies should not be viewed as providing the ultimate criteria for choosing the most clinically significant treatment approach for a given individual case. This can only be done by targeting the particular individual's problem areas, and subsequently using reliable measuring instruments and procedures to determine the patient's response to treatment.

REFERENCES

Burdock, E. I., and Hardesty, A. S. 1967. Childrens Behaviour Inventory. Columbia University, New York. New York State Department of Mental Hygiene.

Conners, C. K., and Eisenberg, L. 1963. The effects of methylphenidate on symptomatology and learning in disturbed children. Am. J. Psychiatry 120:458–464.

Rapoport, J. L., Bucksbaum, M. S., Zahn, P., Wiengartner, H., Ludlaw, C., and Mikkelsen, E. J. 1978. Dextroamaphetamine: Cognitive and behavioral effects in normal prepubertal boys. Science 199:560–563.

Sokolov, E. N. 1963. Perception and the Conditioned Reflex. Macmillan Publishing Company, Inc., New York.

Discussion of "Method and Theory for Psychopharmacology"

Hallgrim Kløve

I certainly found Dr. Conners' orientation toward looking at individual cases very worthwhile. Group studies are of course essential, but it is always nice to go back to the individual, who gives us an opportunity to analyze in detail many of the pitfalls we easily fall into that are not quite appreciated when we are dealing with larger groups.

One of these uncontrolled factors I am thinking about relates to the varying absorption rate of Ritalin, which I feel has been a great source of frustration and has undoubtedly led to many instances of discontinuation of the drug because of inadequate effect.

I wonder also if it is possible at times to account for the difference in behavior in the school situation and at home because the drug has a much greater effect during one part of the day than during another part of the day, a situation that is related to the problems with Ritalin absorption when the drug enters into the intestines. In those cases one might consider the substitution of Ritalin with amphetamine or Cylert. Another area of concern in evaluation of the interaction between the drug and the environment, I think, is how long the child has been on the drug. In using an AB design or variations on this design, I certainly agree with Dr. Kinsbourne's view that with very short medication periods we see a kind of square wave effect. The drug effect tapers off very quickly if the child has been on the drug for a short period, whereas the behavioral changes taper off slowly over several days and even weeks if the child has been on the drug for a longer period of time. In the case studies that Dr. Conners presented, this may be a factor. The duration of drug treatment clearly seems to have a relationship to how long a time it takes for a child to return to baseline after discontinuation of drug treatment. It appears to us that the behavior that we have been trying to eliminate does not recur as quickly when the child has been on drug for a long period of time.

I feel that this represents an interaction with the environment rather than a drug effect alone, since the pharmacological effect of the drug is very short. The explanation is rather that the child has learned to behave in a certain way and that he has also learned to receive various reactions from his environment to his behavior while on drug and this interaction goes on until the child fails in his ability to maintain this system of reinforcement, and the behavior breaks down. For this reason, I feel it is quite important that, when evaluating whether or not a child should continue on medication, a placebo be used. There is a great expectancy factor in the environment dependent on the knowledge about the type of medication the child is receiving. We have often observed that knowledge by others of whether the child is on or off medication determines to an important extent the response to the child. I have often, in individual cases, been impressed with the placebo effect not as much on the child as on the parents or teachers. These observations also emphasize the importance of a comprehensive psychological approach to the treatment of these children in combination with the use of centrally stimulating drugs.

I thought that your observations on the difference in autonomic responses between Dexedrine and amphetamine are extremely interesting and important. In general, it has been assumed that the basic pharmacological effect of the two drugs has been the same, and it may well be that the drugs' effects are the same on central activating mechanisms, but different with regard to peripheral autonomic response patterns. These are observations that are of considerable importance and need to be evaluated further.

Finally, I want to conclude by saying that I am very happy that we have a case study approach represented here. It is very easy to get lost in big groups and the statistics and forget that behind all these numbers and figures are individuals with very heterogeneous problems and complex psychological and neurological interactions. Dr. Conners' papers reminded us again that, although group studies are necessary to get an overview, the individual studies are essential to appreciate the clinical aspects of each single case.

Behavioral Interventions for Hyperactivity

Eric J. Mash
and
J. Thomas Dalby

Research and practice in the areas of behavior therapy and hyperactivity have both accelerated at a remarkable rate over the past 10 years. For behavior therapy this growth is related to its apparent effectiveness in the production of meaningful changes across a wide range of socially relevant behaviors with a relatively minimal amount of professional expense and effort (Franks and Wilson, 1974, 1975, 1976, 1977). The impetus for an increasing interest in hyperactivity is likely related to the now well-documented prevalance of the problem (Lambert, Sandoval, and Sassone, 1977), and to some of the long-term adverse effects associated with this childhood disorder (Mendelson, Johnson, and Stewart, 1971; Weiss et al., 1971; Huessy, Metoyer, and Townsend, 1974).

There is currently some consensus that stimulant medication, particularly methylphenidate and dextroamphetamine, has generally beneficial effects on the behavior of school-age hyperactive children (Sroufe, 1975; Whalen and Henker, 1976; Barkley, 1977; Wolraich, 1977). For example, Gittelman-Klein et al. (1976) state, "no rational, knowledgeable individual can dispute the efficacy of short-term stimulant treatment in the management of hyperactive children." The beneficial effects associated with stimulant medication have been described in a number of excellent reviews (Sroufe, 1975; Barkley, 1977) and include an increased attention span and decreased impulsiveness in responding. However, the use of stimulant medications, as is discussed below, is not without its problems and, consequently, the need for alternative or complementary interventions arises.

Out of the wide array of possible behavioral-psychological-social interventions that may have emerged in this "supplementary" role, behavior therapy seems to have won out as the current nonmedical treatment of choice for hyperactive children (Ross and Ross, 1976). This emergence is based on minimal data that "psychotherapy" is not very effective for hyperactive children (Safer and Allen, 1976) and the need to do something else in those situations where drugs are contraindicated or are partially or totally ineffectual. The emergence of behavior therapy as the most favored treatment is probably a reflection of the fact that both research into hyperactivity and great interest in behavior therapy were occurring at the same time. Although the designation of behavior therapy as the nonmedical treatment of choice for hyperactive children does not rest on a strong empirical base, the small amount of work that has been conducted thus far is promising.

The view of stimulant drugs and behavior therapy as appropriate treatments for hyperactivity has led to the opinion that some combination of the two seems most desirable. Furthermore, individuals responsible for providing help to the hyperactive child and his family should not compete with one another to demonstrate that their method is best. From a research standpoint the questions that have been raised are: 1) is behavior therapy effective in the treatment of hyperactive children; and 2) given that a drug-behavioral treatment is indicated, what are the relative effects associated with the two types of intervention? That is, is one more effective than the other for the same problem? Is one more effective than the other for certain types of problems or in certain situations? Are there interactive effects such that one enhances, facilitates, or has detrimental effects on the action of the other? These questions are dealt with in a later section.

The advocation of a combined behavioral-drug intervention presents behavior therapists with a rather unique situation. There are few, if any, other problem areas in which behavior therapy has been extensively applied where an alternative treatment has been as prevalent and as empirically well documented. Consequently, there has been little comparative research between behavior therapy and other treatments. In addition, the early behavioral stance against a medical model for behavior (Ullman and Krasner, 1965) has led behavior therapists to take a generally antagonistic view toward the use of medical treatments for behavioral problems. Consequently, studies examining behavior-drug effects have been slow in coming and have often been prompted by the fact that the subject or client under study was already on medication, as opposed to being planned out in advance. These issues are implicit in most of the research reviewed in this chapter.

It is the purpose of this chapter to selectively review the research dealing with the application of behavior therapy for the management of hyperactive children and their families. Since the hyperactive child typically exhibits multiple deficits across a wide range of situations, consideration will be given to interventions in a number of settings and for a variety of problems. The review is selective in that it is intended to highlight some of the conceptual and methodological problems that currently exist in the area, and to offer suggestions for future research. Several good reviews of behavioral treatments with hyperactive children are currently available (Simmons, 1975; Ross and Ross, 1976; Safer and Allen, 1976; Ayllon and Rosenbaum, 1977; Brundage-Aguar, Forehand, and Ciminero, 1977; Prout, 1977).

DEFINING BEHAVIOR THERAPY AND HYPERACTIVITY

It is evident that the question, "Is behavior therapy an effective treatment for hyperactivity?" cannot be answered when stated in this global form since it is now well documented that neither behavior therapy (Craighead, Kazdin, and Mahoney, 1976) nor hyperactivity (Langhorne et al., 1976) can be viewed in a unitary fashion. Both terms encompass a heterogeneous set of events, and if our knowledge of the relationship between these sets of events is to be enhanced, it will be necessary to ask questions that are more specific.

The major features of the hyperactive disorder have been well described (Ross and Ross, 1976) and include attentional difficulties, motor activity inappropriate to the situation, impulsivity, distractibility, and irritability.

The occurrence of a range of other problems, including aggression, poor school performance, noncompliance, and difficulties with peers, is also quite common. The scope of problems described by the label is further magnified when one considers the large number of ways each of these broad trait adjectives has been defined and the number of topographically dissimilar behaviors that have been included under such categories as attention and distractibility. The notion that children labeled as hyperactive represent a diverse and heterogeneous group with respect to both symptomatology and probable etiology is commonly accepted. However, despite the fact that several authors have attempted to identify logical groupings of hyperactive children based on etiology (Ney, 1974), empirical efforts to define homogeneous subgroups of hyperactive children based on symptomatology have not been very successful (Langhorne et al., 1976). This heterogeneity has been a persistent problem in investigations of treatment outcome, be they behavior therapy or drugs.

The range of factors encompassed under the "behavior therapy" rubric is formidable. Early treatments of the area tended to view behavior therapy as based on conditioning principles (Wolpe, 1969) and dealing only with observable and overt behavior. Although some continue to adhere to this narrow definition, the more typical view tends to consider conditioning principles only as a loose guideline for conceptualizing behavior and treatments rather than as an explanation for why treatments are effective (Mahoney, Kazdon, and Lesswing, 1974). In part, this shift reflected the fact that many of the things behavior therapists were doing did not seem to follow directly from conditioning paradigms (London, 1972; Krasner, 1976). In addition, the development of cognitive change procedures within a behavior therapy framework (Meichenbaum, 1977) clearly was at odds with a system built on the eschewal of internal events.

Behavior therapy as it has been practiced in treating hyperactive children has included the application of operant programs including positive reinforcement, reinforcement of competing responses, time-out, punishment, extinction, discrimination training, fading and prompting, modeling (Nixon, 1969), instructional materials, cognitive change strategies (including self-instructional training, self-monitoring, and self-reinforcement), token programs, behavioral contracts, relaxation training, biofeedback, role playing, home-based reward systems, parent training, and videotape feedback (Thomas, 1974). This partial list attests to the diversity of interventions that have come to be encompassed under the behavior therapy rubric. This diversity is even greater when one considers that most applications have involved the use of various combinations of the above-mentioned procedures. This "everything but the kitchen sink" picture of behavioral intervention has led some to the conclusion that the term itself has outlived its usefulness (Krasner, 1976). In the present context, however, this state of affairs points up the need to specify exactly what brand of behavior therapy we are practicing in treating hyperactive children. The question then is whether or not a particular procedure is effective for a particular behavior, a statement that may require further qualification in terms of the situation in which the procedure is implemented, by whom, etc. (Kiesler, 1971).

Despite these somewhat muddied waters, there is a set of common features that currently characterize behavior therapy approaches. These include: 1) a commitment to therapy procedures that have some empirical basis; 2) a commitment to a functional analytic approach with the view that our understanding of the causes of behavior and the development of our interventions will best proceed through an identification of those events that immediately precede and follow behavior; and 3) a commitment to an empirical approach to treatment, and specifically to ongoing attempts to objectively document and evaluate the effectiveness of interventions, predominantly through the careful measurement of effects and the utilization of single subject methodology (Sidman, 1960; Hersen and Barlow, 1976).

Behavior therapy approaches are for the most part atheoretical (Risley, 1968), and the application of behavior therapy procedures or the occurrence of successful outcomes do not make any assumptions regarding the etiology of the hyperactive behavior treated. Although some writers have attempted to conceptualize hyperactivity from a learning etiology involving deficient or dysfunctional stimulus control, e.g., as a learned behavior (Willis and Lovaas, 1977), the application of behavior therapy procedures does not imply that the child "learned" to be hyperactive, nor does the successful application of environmental rearrangements to modify behavior imply that some organic dysfunction is not contributing to the occurrence of the behavior. Although etiological information may ultimately serve to guide our intervention efforts, it is currently believed that, given our current state of knowledge, an empirical and pragmatic approach will likely have more immediate benefit. Behavior therapy does assume that contemporaneous environmental events control and influence the occurrence of hyperactive behaviors, a position that even those with a strong leaning toward organic etiology are not likely to take issue with (Wender, 1971).

A RATIONALE FOR BEHAVIORAL INTERVENTION

It is traditional for reviews of this sort (e.g., Brundage-Aguar et al., 1977) and for specific applications of behavior therapy (e.g., Pelham, 1977) to present a rationale for the application of behavioral treatments with hyperactive children in terms of the potential array of limiting conditions associated with the use of stimulant drugs. The voluminous number of limiting conditions that have been identified seems directly proportional to the felt need to convince practitioners that it is reasonable to try something other than psychostimulants in treating hyperactive children. Among the conditions identified are:

1. Drugs may produce a wide range of physical side effects associated with taking stimulant medication, including loss of appetite,

insomnia, weight loss, and irritability (Safer and Allen, 1976; Barkley, 1977). It has been shown that many of these side effects occur more frequently in a group of medicated hyperactive children than in a group of matched controls (Barkley and Cunningham, 1978a).

2. Drugs may produce potentially negative behavioral side effects—for example, reducing the child's social responsiveness (Cunningham and Barkley, 1978; Barkley and Cunningham, 1978a, 1978b), general responsiveness to the environment (Rie et al., 1976a, 1976b), and self-esteem (Campbell, Endman, and Bernfield, 1977).

3. Drug ingestion fails to improve academic performance (Allen, 1977; Barkley and Cunningham, 1978c).

4. Taking drugs may adversely affect the attributional system of the child (Whalen and Henker, 1976).

5. Learning that occurs while the child is medicated may be temporary (Rie and Rie, 1977), in that it may be either state dependent (Swanson and Kinsbourne, 1976) or a discriminated operant with drug state as the discriminative cue (Colpaert, 1977).

6. Parents may resist the use of medication.

7. Drugs may suggest to the parent or teacher than the child is being adequately treated and that it is not necessary to do anything else (Rie and Rie, 1977).

8. The long-term effects of drug ingestion are not clear and there is some indication that children who are on medication do not ultimately do better than those who are not.

9. Some children, approximately 20%–30%, do not respond to medication.

10. Drug effects may not be evident in the relatively unstructured home situation.

11. For many children hyperactivity may not be related to organic dysfunction (Dubey, 1976; Rutter, 1977). This rationale implies that if there is no organic dysfunction then there is no basis for assuming that drugs will have beneficial effects.

Although there likely will be disagreement and conflicting evidence regarding the validity of these points, it is nevertheless the case that all of them have been presented in support of the utilization of behavior therapy procedures. However, although the above-mentioned factors may very well support the notion that under certain conditions drugs should not be used, none of them provides a specific rationale for the utilization of behavior therapy in contrast to any other therapeutic alternative. The rationale for the utilization of a behavioral approach to the treatment of hyperactive children should come from a more positive source rather than being dependent on purported limitations of drug treatment. The logical candidates would be rationales based on theory, practice, and empirical support.

An excellent elaboration of the conceptual rationale for the use of behavior therapy with hyperactive children was presented by Werry and Sprague (1970). Unfortunately, in the furor that followed this paper many of the important points seem to have been lost. These authors described hyperactivity as a behavioral disorder that results in conflict with the social environment because of its inappropriateness to the situation. Since the nature of the disorder is in part social, the need to consider interventions that take such factors into account is evident. Werry and Sprague also review a number of potential advantages of behavioral treatments. The approach is problem oriented and therefore more likely to be perceived as meaningful by those complaining, with a consequent increase in their willingness to cooperate during treatment. This point receives some support from a study by Dubey, Kaufman, and O'Leary (1977a, 1977b) in which a behavioral approach to training parents of hyperactive children was compared with a relationship-oriented approach (PET; Gordon, 1970). Parents in the behavioral group felt that the course was more applicable to their problems and were less likely to drop out of treatment.

A second advantage of behavior modification described by Werry and Sprague is that, because of the emphasis on behavior rather than mental or mediating responses, the approach is particularly suited to the treatment of young children and behaviors for which verbal persuasion has not been effective. This point no longer seems relevant. The trend in behavior therapy has been toward an increasing recognition and emphasis on the role of cognitive events in mediating behavior change (Meichenbaum, 1977). Historically, behavioral treatments with hyperactive children have not been with children who were preverbal, but rather more with school-age populations.

A third point made by Werry and Sprague is that the experimental roots of behavior therapy make it an approach that is more likely to lead to assessments of therapy and adequate research. There is no question that behavioral interventions have consistently attempted to assess therapy outcomes. Whether or not these attempts have constituted adequate research is a question that is considered later in this chapter.

Finally, Werry and Sprague state that the explicitness of behavior therapy procedures permits their implementation by relatively unskilled persons such as child care workers, students, teachers, and parents, thus constituting a relatively rich source of manpower. Behavioral treatments with hyperactive children have in fact been carried out by a wide range of individuals, as predicted; however, this application by nonprofessionsls has at times led to misuse (Bachrach.and Quigley, 1966) and abuse (Goldiamond, 1974).

To summarize the major points by Werry and Sprague, behavior therapy has promise since it deals with a social problem with a social solution (the labeling of hyperactivity as a social problem does not imply that the etiology is social, only that social factors are inextricably involved), uses methods that are self-evaluating, is relevant to the specific problems and concerns expressed by parents and teachers and is therefore likely to be used, and is economical and feasible since it has the prospect of meeting the needs of hyperactive children through the use of relevant nonprofessionals. These points provide a conceptual rationale for using behavior therapy that does not depend on the limiting conditions of stimulant medication. Of course, a rationale based on empirical effectiveness is the strongest one for the utilization of behavioral procedures. The basis for such utilization is considered in the remainder of this chapter.

REINFORCEMENT APPLICATIONS IN THE LABORATORY

Several laboratory investigations have examined the responses of hyperactive children to varying conditions of reward. A number of these studies suggest that hyperactive children respond to reinforcement contingencies in unique ways (Douglas, 1975). Hyperactive children may become overinvolved in the reinforcers or reinforcing agent and show deterioration in performance under random or partial reinforcement conditions (Freibergs and Douglas, 1969; Parry and Douglas, 1973). It has also been demonstrated that the performance of hyperactive children quickly returns to baseline following the termination of reinforcement, e.g., extinction, and frustration is evident (Cohen, 1970; Parry and Douglas, 1973), and that hyperactive children may show a deterioration in performance related to shifts in self-reinforcement schedules (Barkley, Copeland, and Sivage, 1978). The above findings would suggest that reward programs should begin with continuous and contingent reinforcement, removal of which should be done gradually. Douglas (1972) proposes that the child might be taught to administer his own rewards, thus making reinforcement partially independent of outside agents. This approach would be consistent with the many reports demonstrating the efficacy of self-reinforcement programs (Mahoney, 1974; Thoreson and Mahoney, 1974; Barkley et al., 1978; Varni and Henker, in press).

Firestone and Douglas (1975) compared the performance of hyperactive and control children on a reaction-time task under reward, punishment, and reward plus punishment conditions. All three conditions resulted in improved performance for both groups, but the reward only condition led to a significant increase in impulsive responses for hyperactive children. The hyperactive children exhibited less impulsivity with mildly negative feedback. Firestone and Douglas (1977) also reported that cognitively impulsive children performed more poorly than reflective subjects under reward, but not under punishment, conditions.

Worland (1976) found that, although positive and negative feedback conditions reduced off-task behavior in hyperactive children, negative feedback resulted in a decrease in the accuracy of their performances on a spelling correction task. The subjects were punished for off-task behaviors and not for task performance. As Ayllon and Roberts (1974) have noted, reinforcing children for increasing their on-task behavior does not necessarily increase their task performance. This suggests that reinforcement and punishment should be directly related to the behavior desired, rather than used indirectly for behaviors that are assumed to lead to this terminal response. Both studies investigating punishment (Firestone and Douglas, 1975; Worland, 1976) with hyperactive children found it to be an effective technique. However, as Worland quite appropriately suggests, the potential side effects must be carefully evaluated before any punishment procedure is used.

Although the internal validity of these laboratory investigations is possibly high, the degree to which we can generalize these findings to behavior therapy applications is questionable. The findings are severely restricted by the specific response measures, the types of reinforcers, and the parameters of reinforcement utilized. They do, however, offer useful suggestions for areas that require further empirical investigation under more naturalistic circumstances. The suggestion that hyperactive children respond to reinforcement contingencies in "unique" ways has led some investigators to a skeptical view of intervention strategies with hyperactive children based exclusively on contingency management (Douglas et al., 1976). However, the evidence in support of the view that hyperactive children are unique in their reactions to reinforcement is minimal, and the number of successful applications of reinforcement programs with hyperactives suggests a fairly predictable response to reinforcement (Ross and Ross, 1976). It is also unlikely that the reinforcement conditions utilized in the laboratory studies described directly parallel the range and combination of contingency management procedures used in the actual treatment of hyperactive children. These findings do, however, suggest the need for a careful assessment with any given child of the real effects of the various reinforcement operations that might be employed, and indicate some of the problems involved in assuming that particular stimulus events always operate as reinforcers or punishers.

REINFORCEMENT TECHNIQUES

The use of reinforcement techniques to alter hyperactive behavior was initially reported by Patterson (Patterson, 1965; Patterson et al., 1965). His experimental subjects (N = 1 for both studies) were described as brain damaged, academically retarded, and adopted, therefore limiting generalization of the findings to hyperactive children per se. In both of these studies, using candy as reinforcement, hyperactive movement was decreased. Follow-up (4-month telephone follow-up; 4-week extinction period) indicated that behavior change had been maintained. Douglas (1974) points out, however, that there is no evidence that a reduction in activity level is accompanied by improved learning.

Doubros and Daniels (1966) implemented a token reinforcement program with six overactive mentally retarded children. They successfully reduced both verbal and motor overactivity in the classroom and the effect persisted during a 1-week extinction phase and 1 week thereafter.

Pihl (1967) presented two case reports, one with a retarded subject and one with a brain-damaged subject, both reportedly hyperactive. Using token reinforcement, both subjects reduced the amount of time they moved from a chair placed in an empty room. Success in generalizing this program to behaviors in the home was claimed in one case.

Using adults' social reinforcement, Allen et al. (1967) successfully managed the hyperactive, inattentive behavior of a 4½-year-old boy. Anecdotal reports by the mother indicated that the treatment effects generalized to the home. Their procedures increased attending behavior, but did not generalize to social behavior.

Twardosz and Sajwaj (1972) used a prompting and differential reinforcement procedure to increase sitting in a 4-year-old hyperactive retarded boy in a remedial preschool. Unlike the previous study, however, desirable collateral changes such as use of toys and proximity to other children increased. No follow-up information was provided.

Using a home-based reinforcement program, O'Leary et al. (1976) sought to increase academic and prosocial behavior for nine hyperactive boys. Their study was superior in several respects to other efforts: 1) use of individualized reinforcements; 2) use of a control group; and 3) use of parents as reinforcing agents. Although the authors report probabilities in their results, no statistics were presented and no follow-up data were reported.

Rosenbaum, O'Leary, and Jacob (1975) found that both individualized and group rewards were effective in reducing hyperactive behavior as measured by the Conners Teacher Rating Scale. The group reward program was significantly more popular with the teachers than was the individualized reward program. This indicated to the authors that such group interventions are indicated, because a popular program not only has a greater probability of being used, but once used has a higher probability of being maintained.

Alabiso (1975) used token and social reinforcement to increase attention in eight institutionalized hyperactive retardates. He measured sitting behavior, digit copying, and discrimination learning under different reinforcement schedules, with the result that correct responses increased with increases in the response-reinforcement ratio. Taken together, the reinforcement studies described are limited by their use of few subjects and atypical populations, their choice of dependent measures, and their failure to obtain adequate follow-up information. These problems are further discussed later in the chapter.

COMPARISONS OF DRUG AND BEHAVIORAL INTERVENTIONS

The prevalent use of stimulant medication along with the increasing applications of behavior therapy as an adjunct or alternative in the treatment of hyperactive children has led to an increasing interest in studies comparing the two approaches. In considering the somewhat illegitimate relationship between drugs and behavior therapy, several authors (Eysenck and Rachman, 1971; Sprague and Werry, 1971) have attempted to legitimize it by alluding to the possibility that drugs may serve to enhance conditionability and consequently might facilitate behavior therapy efforts. Also, the child may be quieted by medication, which then permits the learning of more appropriate behaviors. However, there is currently no direct support for the notion that stimulants facilitate operant conditioning in hyperactive children (Gittelman-Klein et al., 1976). In addition, it is possible that reverse effects might occur; that is, the child may be less responsive to *certain types of behavioral interventions* when medicated. For example, if medication does reduce social responsiveness and increase solitary play, as noted by some authors (Schleifer et al., 1975; Barkley and Cunningham, 1978a, 1978c), then it may serve to reduce the effectiveness of procedures based on social reinforcement or oriented toward teaching appropriate social skills.

Direct comparisons of the relative and combined effects of stimulant drug and behavioral management treatments have been few. Christensen and Sprague (1973) investigated the effects of conditioning procedures alone and in combination with methylphenidate, with seat movement as the dependent variable. Their drug-plus-conditioning group ($N = 6$) displayed rates of movement that were consistently lower than their conditioning-only group ($N = 6$). In addition, the drug-plus-conditioning group maintained their low rate of movement after reinforcement contingencies were withdrawn, whereas the other group showed an immediate increase in movement.

Several problems limit the generality of these findings. First, the dependent measure, seat movement, has a dubious relationship to the central attentional dysfunction of this population (Douglas, 1972; Ross, 1976). Second, the criterion for reinforcement in the study was based on initial level of performance. Since the nonmedicated group had higher activity measures initially, they presumably could earn the same amount of reinforcement while responding at higher levels. It is not clear from the study whether there were any differences in the amount of reinforcement that was received by children in the two groups.

Ayllon, Layman, and Kandel (1975) reported academic and behavioral improvement using contingency management techniques with three children who had previously been taking stimulants. However, the drug dosages their subjects had been receiving were much lower than the mean dosage usually found to be clinically effective with children this age (Barkley, 1977). Although it is recognized that the dosage appropriate for a particular subject is idiosyncratic, it is improbable that all three children would need such a low dosage. Hence, it is questionable whether or not the medication baseline can be critically compared to results obtained with the reinforcement procedure. Other drawbacks of the study were the limited sample size and the lack of any follow-up information. Although these results are promising, further research with more children examining long-term effects is needed. The authors' inclusion of academic measures along with behavioral ratings was a notable feature of this study.

In another study examining drug versus reinforcement procedures with a single hyperactive child, Wulbert and Dries (1977) compared performance across settings and tasks. In the clinic setting their subject displayed no significant drug effects, but drug effects were noted within the home. Reinforcement contingencies were successful in the clinic but did not generalize to the home. There was a particular emphasis on the subject's ritualistic behavior, which is not typical of hyperactive children. In addition, no follow-up was provided. Their study does alert us to the need to monitor stimulus and response generalization of treatment effects.

Another single-subject study comparing medication and contingency management (Shafto and Sulzbacher, 1977) found that fewer free play activity changes occurred during contingency phases. Medication increased attention more at low doses. Their subject's speech before the study was predominantly echoic, and he had been referred with a diagnosis of mental retardation. Hyperactive children, despite their attentional dysfunction, obtain at least normal IQs on standardized tests, hence, this subject is not typical of children referred for hyperactivity. In addition, the changes were short term and not maintained.

Pelham (1976, 1977) used a home-based reinforcement program in combination with parent training to control the hyperactive behavior of a 9-year-old boy. The program was instituted while the boy was receiving medication and after 7 weeks the medication was withdrawn. Behavior change was measured by teacher and parent ratings. Methodological problems included a lack of a baseline with no intervention. In this study, it is not possible to assess the relative benefits, if any, of the treatments. It may have been that the child was responding adversely to medical intervention and would have improved simply by withdrawing it.

One of the better controlled studies on the effects of stimulant medication and behavior modification on hyperactive children (Gittelman-Klein et al., 1976) found that the groups receiving methylphenidate improved significantly more on behavior ratings than the group receiving behavior therapy alone. No significant differences were found between the methylphenidate alone and methylphenidate combined with behavior therapy groups. The relatively large sample size ($N = 34$), in addition to the superior design, increases the importance of this ongoing study, which is discussed again later in the chapter.

Wolraich et al. (1978) compared the effects of methylphenidate alone and in combination with behavior modification procedures on the classroom behaviors and academic performances of hyperactive children. The relative effectiveness of behavior modification and medication was related to the period during which behavior was observed, with the token economy having generally beneficial effects in a group work situation and medication having positive effects during individual work time. Behavior modification alone significantly affected academic performance. It should be pointed out that the generality of these findings are limited to the extent that the program was carried out over a short period of time (6 weeks), and no follow-up data are presented.

Christensen (1975) examined the effects of combining stimulant treatment with a classroom token system for 13 hyperactive retarded children. Using multiple measures (movement, ratings, academic performance, and observations) he found that a token reinforcement program with placebo resulted in significant overall improvement. The addition of stimulant medication resulted in no further improvement. No trial of stimulant alone was given and the nature of his subjects limits the comparison value of the study.

Comparison studies of drugs and behavior modification can be improved in several ways. First, it must be established whether a subject is favorably or adversely responsive to stimulant medication. This would eliminate a partial cancellation of positive treatment effects. Second, individual dosages must be clinically titrated for those who respond favorably. It is well known that psychotropic drug schedules are extremely idiosyncratic with children, and the use of fixed dosages or dosages based on subjects' weights are not clinically effective. Such drug adjustments should, however, take place prior to the introduction of other interventions. More adequate baselines, follow-up, and generalization data are needed in future drug–behavior therapy comparisons.

COGNITIVE BEHAVIOR MODIFICATION

There has been a recent shift in behavior therapy toward the use of more cognitively oriented interventions in the treatment of behavior disorders (Mahoney, 1974; Meichenbaum, 1974, 1977; Goldfried and Davison, 1976). Particular emphasis has been given to the development of self-regulatory processes (Kanfer and Karoly, 1972), including self-observation, self-monitoring, and self-reinforcement (Goldfried and Merbaum, 1974; Thoreson and Mahoney, 1974; Bandura, 1977). Cognitive change procedures for hyperactive children have followed from the self-instructional approach described in several early studies (Palkes, Stewart, and Kahana, 1968; Meichenbaum and Goodman, 1969a, 1969b, 1971). The rationale presented for the use of self-control strategies with hyperactive children is:

1. Self-control training targets the qualitative deficits specific to this population, including an inability to inhibit activity when the situation calls for it, an overly impulsive response style, and the lack of a careful and deliberate approach to the solution of problems. With this approach, attentional deficits are assumed to be primary and the assumption is that if they can be overcome, secondary problems such as academic failure or social difficulty will also change. Con-

sequently, the approach assumes that response generalization will occur.

2. If the performance of the child can be brought under "internal" or self-control, the likelihood that behavior change will generalize across situations and across time is increased, since performance is not dependent on the presence of extrinsic cues or reinforcers.

3. Increasing self-control may alter self-perception and increase self-esteem (Bugental, Whalen, and Henker, 1977).

Palkes et al. (1968) were the first to experimentally implement self-instruction with hyperactive children. Their work was based on earlier suggestions by Luria (1961). Twenty hyperactive boys of normal intelligence were divided into an experimental and a control group. After only two 30-minute training sessions the experimental group improved significantly on the Porteus Mazes and the control group did not. The posttest was administered immediately after the second training session and no follow-up or generalization information was obtained.

A later study (Palkes, Stewart, and Freedman, 1972) examined the effects of silently read versus vocalized self-directed commands. With 10 subjects in each of these experimental conditions and an additional 10 subjects as controls, they again used the Porteus Mazes in a pre-post design. They found that the group trained to vocalize commands improved significantly and the other groups did not. This improvement, however, did not extend to performance 2 weeks later. The authors suggested that repeated training sessions be utilized to prolong treatment effects.

Meichenbaum and Goodman (1969a, 1969b, 1971) have also explored verbal control of children's behavior. In the 1971 study, five impulsive children were trained to talk to themselves, initially overtly and then covertly, in an attempt to increase self-directed control. They found improvement, after four ½-hour training sessions, on the performance scale of the WISC, the Porteus Mazes, and the Matching Familiar Figures Test (MFFT). It is questionable whether or not these children can be considered "hyperactive" because they were selected from an "opportunity remedial class" that contained a heterogeneous group of behavior problems. Although improvement on the experimental measures was maintained at the 4-week follow-up, the treatment effects did not generalize to the classroom. Despite difficulties in the study, Meichenbaum and Goodman's work inspired a number of later investigations evaluating self-instructional procedures with hyperactive children and other atypical populations.

Bornstein and Quevillon (1976) investigated the effects of self-instruction on three overactive preschool boys. The dependent measure was "on-task" behavior, which was assessed by two naïve judges. After a 2-hour training period, there was an immediate and dramatic increase in on-task behavior. The strengths of this study included using a multiple baseline design across subjects and the presentation of long-term follow-up data. In addition, it was found that treatment effects generalized from experimental tasks to the classroom. The findings of this study, however, have not been replicated (O'Leary, 1977).

Burns (1972) assigned 45 urban school-age hyperactives to either an experimental group receiving 20 trials in self-verbalization, a group receiving 40 trials, or a control group. The dependent measures were arithmetic performance and activity level. The training procedure had no beneficial effects.

Douglas et al. (1976) studied the effects of modeling, self-verbalization, and self-reinforcement techniques on hyperactive boys. Eighteen subjects were placed in a training group and eleven boys were placed in a control group. The training period was much more extensive than in other studies, covering a 3-month period in which the children were seen for two 1-hour sessions per week for a total of 24 sessions. In addition, six sessions were held with the child's teacher and 12 with parents to discuss the treatment program. The dependent measure was a comprehensive battery of cognitive and motor tasks. Improvement was noted on half of the measures and these were generally maintained. It was interesting that the two measures used by Burns (1972), arithmetic and motor activity, also failed to improve in this study. Douglas et al. explain the lack of change on the Conners Teacher Rating Scale by the fact that their training program stressed internal thought processes and the development of inner controls far more heavily than outwardly observed behavior, and, with time, it is possible that delayed effects might "take hold." Such a view is somewhat at odds with the response generalization assumption frequently made in self-instructional programs, and the evidence for "delayed effects" in behavior therapy programs is minimal. It was not possible to isolate specific variables that influenced the children's performance because of their multiple treatment approach. Their study, however, is an example of a comprehensive clinical research program derived from the findings of previous experimental investigations.

In a recent study, Barkley et al., (1978) designed a classroom situation for six hyperactive boys in which self-instruction, self-monitoring, and self-reinforcement were utilized. A comprehensive assessment battery was utilized to evaluate the outcome. In general, the self-control package was effective in reducing misbehavior and improving task attention; however, classroom performance was only minimally affected by the intervention. The authors suggest that interventions over time periods longer than the 8 weeks of this study may be necessary if changes in academic performance are to be produced. In addition, there were no generalized effects to nontreatment settings.

In a well-controlled within-subject design, Varni and Henker (in press) trained three hyperactive disruptive boys utilizing a self-regulation approach including self-instruction, self-monitoring, and self-reinforcement. Hyperactive behaviors and academic performance during reading and math were monitored in both school and clinic settings. Verbal self-instructional training did not result in improved performance in the absence of adult supervision, and self-monitoring had little effect. A combination of self-monitoring and self-reinforcement techniques introduced first in the clinic and then in the school resulted in increases in academic performance with concomitant reductions in hyperactive behaviors. This study is important in identifying the components of self-control strategies that may be necessary in producing change and because of the demonstrable effects on academic performance. The findings of this study are consistent with others in pointing up the importance of including a self-reinforcement component in cognitive change programs (Barkley et al., 1978).

A number of authors have used instruction in self-verbalizations with other atypical child populations, such as emotionally disturbed boys (Finch et al., 1975; Kendall and Finch, 1976, 1978), and young aggressive boys (Camp et al., 1977), with some favorable results.

Bender (1976) notes that verbal self-instruction taught in conjunction with task-specific strategies may be more adaptive than simply trying to modify latency of response in hyperactive children. As Zivin (1974) points out, slowing action tempo may or may not be an important step toward reducing performance errors. Dalby et al. (1977) focused on system change rather than target change and found that performance on a learning task with hyperactive children was best when items to be learned were presented at a brisk pace. In conditions where longer intervals were available to study, performance deteriorated. Hence, slowing cognitive tempo may not be adaptive in all situations.

In learning situations with normal populations, tempo is usually slow when material is unfamiliar, but once strategies are mastered tempo quickens. With the hyperactive child, slowing cognitive tempo in new learning situations and teaching task-specific strategies may be useful. Once a task is familiar, however, continued slow pacing may be detrimental. Self-pacing may be more adaptive at this point (Dalby et al., 1977).

Although preliminary work with self-instructional training is encouraging, the findings from many of the studies described have not always been replicable (Higa, 1973; Mash and Sinclair, 1977; O'Leary, 1977). There is little support for the assumption that teaching self-control generalizes to performance on non–training tasks, and minimal evidence thus far for the generality of self-control training across situations or over long periods of time. In addition, the data do not support the assumption that increases in self-control will be accompanied by changes in self-concept. In fact, one study (Kendall and Finch, 1978) found no changes in self-perceptions of impulsivity for emotionally disturbed children, in spite of the fact that impulsivity changes were noted in test performance. Finally, where self-instruction has been employed the training package is quite complex, often including modeling, self-instructions, self-reinforcement, response-cost, etc. There is a need to identify which aspect of the program might be contributing most to change (Kendall, 1977).

PROGRESSIVE RELAXATION AND BIOFEEDBACK TRAINING

Putre et al. (1977) used progressive relaxation training with 20 hyperactive boys in a treatment center for emotionally disturbed and socially maladjusted children. Half of the boys received sessions where they listened to a tape of systematic instructions to alternately tense and relax muscles. The other group listened to tapes of stories read from boys' adventure books. Both groups significantly decreased average frontalis muscle tension after 2 weeks of training, suggesting that any effects were not specific to relaxation training. In addition, physiological changes were not related to behavioral measures.

Nall (1973) attempted alpha-training with hyperkinetic children; however, the results of this study were inconclusive. In another study, Simpson and Nelson (1972) gave children exhibiting hyperactive behavior feedback regarding their breathing rate. Experimental subjects showed reductions in breathing irregularity, better task performance, and increased attention. However, these changes occurred only in the training sessions, with no transfer to other situations.

Other studies (Braud, 1975; Braud, Lupin, and Braud, 1975; Haight, Irvine, and Jampolsky, 1976) have reported the use of frontalis electromyographic (EMG) biofeedback with hyperactive children and have reported general improvements in the children's attentional abilities and test performances. However, these studies did not relate their results to observable classroom behavior. Bryant and Hunter (1977) attempted to do this with 20 school-age children described as "severe attention problems" by their teachers. Both biofeedback and pseudobiofeedback subjects learned to lower frontalis EMG levels, with a greater reduction for biofeedback subjects. However, these changes were not related to improvements in the children's abilities to focus attention or to spend more time on task in the classroom. The authors suggest that some additional environment cueing may be necessary to get children to use the skill they have learned. As previously mentioned, similar approaches might be useful in relation to self-control training strategies.

Lubar and Shouse (1976, 1977) have reported the use with hyperactive children of biofeedback involving conditioning of sensorimotor rhythm (SMR). A subgroup of children who exhibited SMR in the 4–7 Hz range were trained in the production of SMR in the 12–14 Hz range and inhibition of rhythms in the 4–7 Hz range. This subgroup of children was also noted to be more responsive to stimulant medication prior to training. The training resulted in significant physiological changes in the lab and behavioral change in other settings. It was noted that combining medication and SMR conditioning led to greater change in hyperkinetic behaviors than the use of drugs alone, and benefit of the SMR training was maintained following the withdrawal of medication. The findings from this research are intriguing, but require further replication with larger numbers of subjects. Although biofeedback training with some subcategories of hyperactive children would appear to have promise, future research should give careful attention to some of the conceptual and methodological concerns that have been raised about the use of biofeedback generally (Black and Cott, 1977).

CLASSROOM INTERVENTIONS

Behavioral classroom interventions with hyperactive children have been reviewed in detail elsewhere (Ayllon and Rosenbaum, 1977) and are only mentioned briefly. The prevalence of classroom difficulties for hyperactives requires that any therapeutic program consider behavior in the school setting. The effectiveness of behavioral techniques in modifying "disruptive" behavior in the classroom is well documented (O'Leary and O'Leary, 1972). Specific behaviors described as disruptive have included inappropriate vocalization, aggression toward peers, talking out, and out-of-seat and off-task behavior. Together, these behaviors have been called "inattentive" (Kazdin, 1973), or "study" behavior (Hall, Lund, and Jackson, 1968). One must be cautious, however, in viewing reductions in disruptive classroom behavior as successful demonstrations of behavioral procedures with hyperactive children (Ayllon, Layman, and Kandel, 1975).

Given that the primary goal in the classroom situation is effective learning, investigators have assumed that, for hyperactive children, a reduction in the inattentive disruptive behaviors described previously will lead to enhanced learning. However, the evidence in support of this notion is minimal. Ayllon and Rosenbaum (1977) have suggested that programs that directly alter academic performance will serve to reduce disruptive behavior (Ayllon, Layman, and Burke, 1972; Ayllon and Roberts, 1974; Ayllon, Layman, and Kandel, 1975). If academic performance represents the terminal link in a behavioral chain, then presumably competing inattentive and disruptive behaviors will drop out as academic performance increases. The results of the research by Ayllon and his colleagues offer some support for this notion. In any case, behavioral interventions clearly need to focus more on academic targets in the future, rather than focusing exclusively on the reduction of disruptive responding. Adequate data on the usefulness of behavioral strategies in modifying the academic performance of hyperactive children are not yet available, although several studies (Ayllon, Layman, and Kandel, 1975; Varni and Henker, in press; Wolraich et al., 1978) indicate promise.

More attention needs to be given to the role of the hyperactive child as part of a larger classroom system. Direct observations of classroom interactions between hyperactive children and their peers, similar to those reported by Campbell et al. (1977), are needed. More attention should also be directed to the relationship between classroom and home programs, and the generalization of effects across settings needs to be considered, especially in light of the cross-setting interventions (i.e., home-based reinforcement) that have been used (Bailey, Wolf, and Phillips, 1970; Ayllon, Garber, and Pisor, 1975; O'Leary et al., 1976).

It is likely that behavioral interventions will receive increased use in the classroom in light of the fact that drug interventions alone have not been shown to have much of an effect on academic performance (Barkley and Cunningham, 1978b). In assessing the relative effects of drugs and behavioral interventions in the classroom, however, it will be important to consider the effects of drug dose (Sprague and Sleator, 1977) and classroom activity (Wolraich et al., 1978).

BEHAVIORAL INTERVENTION WITH FAMILIES

The conceptual rationale and procedures for behavioral intervention with families have been fully described (Mash, Hamerlynck, and Handy, 1976; Mash, Handy, and Hamerlynck, 1976). Specifically, the family focus in behavior therapy recognizes the role of family factors in the development and maintenance of disturbed behavior, as well as the role of the disturbed behavior in affecting the entire family system (Patterson, 1976). If the problem is to be eliminated, changes must occur in the entire family system. In addition, limited manpower combined with the large number of disturbed children needing assistance makes the utilization of family members as resource individuals an economically viable alternative to intervention by professionals (Tharp and Wetzel, 1969). There are several reasons that interventions with the families of hyperactive children seem important. In addition to school difficulties, hyperactive children frequently exhibit behavior problems in the home, including irritability, noncompliance, and aggression and are difficult to manage. Parents' perceptions of the problem and how they ultimately deal with it are likely to affect long-term outcomes (Loney, Comly, and Simon, 1975), and possibly the child's response to stimulant medication (Conrad and Insel, 1967; Barkley and Cunningham, 1978c). There is also evidence that the presence of a disturbed child in the system is related to problems in other family members (Arnold, Levine, and Patterson, 1975), particularly siblings (Mash and Mercer, 1979).

Several authors have outlined a behavioral approach to managing the hyperactive child and have recognized both the need to intervene in several settings (e.g., clinic, classroom, and home), and the importance of involving and training family members (Feighner, 1975; Simmons, 1975; Willis and Lovaas, 1977; Pelham, 1978). These discussions are typically supported by anecdotal material and case reports. There has recently been an increase in the number of studies that have attempted to utilize and systematically evaluate behavior therapy procedures with families. Typically such interventions have been implemented across several settings (Feighner and Feighner, 1974) or in combination with medication (Gittelman-Klein et al., 1976) or clinic training (Douglas et al., 1976) and it is not possible to evaluate the separate impact of family intervention apart from the total program.

Several studies have reported the use of group counseling sessions with parents in which behavior modification principles are discussed as they apply to common problems, and parents work at modifying specific target behaviors (Feighner and Feighner, 1974; Gittelman-Klein and Klein, 1975; Dubey et al., 1977a, 1977b; O'Leary and Pelham, 1978). Dubey et al. (1977b) provided parents of hyperactive children with 2-hour weekly meetings over a period of 9 weeks that involved reading, lecture-discussions, and homework that included observation and recording of parent and child behavior and the implementation of change programs. The emphasis was on teaching parents general skills. The program was evaluated utilizing multiple measures and, in comparison with a no-treatment control group, significant changes were noted on parent ratings of hyperactivity (Werry-Weiss-Peters scale) and global improvement, but not on laboratory observations of behavior. It was also found that parents trained to utilize a relationship-oriented approach (PET; Gordon, 1970) showed similar changes, but were more likely to drop out and less likely to recommend the program to a friend. Although this study is a significant improvement over the anecdotal accounts and case reports of behavior training with parents, there were a number of limitations, including the possibility that the treatment and control groups were not equivalent, the unequal numbers of parents in each group, and the absence of any follow-up information. The differences in outcome as assessed by the various dependent measures point up the need to utilize multiple outcome assessments in evaluating behavior interventions with parents of hyperactive children.

Wulbert and Dries (1977) described the use of a mother-administered token economy in the home with a 9-year-old hyperactive boy. The child was given points for cooperative behavior and compliance and was placed in time-out for aggressive behavior (Sachs, 1973). The mother also collected data on the child's ritualistic, distractible, and aggressive behavior. Concomitant with the home program, the child was involved in twice-weekly clinic sessions in which he was reinforced for performance on visual and auditory tasks. The child also received medication or placebo in a double-blind design over the 8 weeks. In the home setting, the child showed an increase in ritualistic behavior but a decrease in aggressive behavior when on Ritalin as compared with placebo. However, since several programs were being carried out simultaneously, it is difficult to assess the specific contribution of the home program to any changes that may have occurred. The fact that aggression in the home was related to medication status rather than time in the program suggests that the home reinforcement procedures may not have been effective or that they were only effective when the child was medicated. In addition, no follow-up data were presented, and changes in the home were monitored exclusively through the observations by the mother with no reliability information presented.

Pelham (1976, 1977) described the implementation of a behavioral intervention program in the school and home for a 9-year-old hyperkinetic boy, with the concomitant withdrawal of stimulant medication. The parents were seen 14 times over a 7-month period and a concurrent school program was carried out. The parent training focused on teaching contingency management skills through discussion, readings, and observation of videotaped structured interaction involving the child, his parents, and sibling. The teacher was instructed in the use of contingency management skills, and a home-based reward program following that described by O'Leary et al. (1976) was instituted in which the child earned money for positive reports from school. Both teacher and parent ratings of hyperactivity decreased over the course of treatment and continued to do so following the withdrawal of medication. While the change in teacher ratings resulted in a post-therapy score within the normal range for the Conners Abbreviated Teacher Rating Scale (CATRS; Sprague, Cohen, and Werry, 1974), the post-treatment rating by parents was still well above age norms (Routh, Schroeder, and O'Tuama, 1974).

An 11-month follow-up contact showed a slight reduction in parent ratings, although still well above age norm, and an increased CATRS rating by the child's next grade teacher. There are numerous problems with this case study, including a lack of adequate controls, subjective ratings of change combined with an awareness by the parents and teachers of changes in medication, subjective and partially noncomparable follow-up measures, and simultaneous interventions across settings. All of these factors call into question whether or not the changes reported were reliable or significant, and if they were attributable to the behavioral interventions. The study does, however, describe some of the frequently used behavioral interventions with families.

One of these, videotape feedback to parents of hyperactive children, has been described in a number of reports (Furman and Feighner, 1973; Feighner, 1975; Pelham, 1977). Although the procedure appears to have promise in assisting parents in identifying and tracking the interactions between themselves and their children, and as a vehicle for teaching reinforcement principles, it has not been systematically evaluated. Mash and McElwee (1978) reported changes in behavior relative to a control condition following group training that included videotape feedback for parents of children who exhibited a range of behavior problems including hyperactivity. The changes that occurred were not specific to whether parents observed themselves interacting with their child or another parent-child dyad. Unfortunately, it was not possible to assess the specific effects of the videotape feedback, since it was utilized in conjunction with other interventions, including home observation, didactic sessions, reading materials, and parent-child contracts. The use of multiple interventions across multiple settings for many hyperactive children makes it difficult to isolate specific treatment effects. In any case, videotape feedback with parents of hyperactive children is an approach that has promise but requires further empirical study.

A number of investigators (O'Leary et al., 1976; Pelham, 1977) have attempted to bridge the gap between school and home treatment of hyperactive children through the use of home-based reinforcement systems either alone (O'Leary et al., 1976) or in conjunction with other reinforcement procedures in the classroom. The procedure involves the child receiving a report to be taken home that indicates whether or not the child has met some behavioral criteria, and if so, he is rewarded by the parents. This procedure has been used effectively in promoting both academic and nonacademic behaviors in the classroom.

O'Leary et al. (1976) used such a procedure over a 10-week period to treat children rated as hyperactive by both parents and teachers. Academic and prosocial behaviors were targeted for change in the classroom, in contrast to many interventions in which attending, sitting still, and fidgeting have been selected as the treatment focus. Following treatment, the teacher ratings of hyperactivity for the nine children receiving the home-based program showed a significant decline and were lower than ratings for a control group. Noteworthy in this study was an initial attempt to establish an independent validation of teacher ratings through comparisons with direct observations of classroom behavior. Unfortunately, such observations were not made following treatment and the outcome is limited in its use of only subjective verbal report measures that are likely influenced by the teacher's awareness of the child's participation in the home-based reward program. Rather than a no-treatment control, a more adequate test might be one in which the control group children were given home reports but parents were not instructed to act on them. In such a program, teachers could not readily discriminate which children were being "treated" and which were not, thus reducing the probability of obtaining biased ratings. This study also does not include any post-treatment measures of the child's behavior in the home. Parent rating scales (Werry-Weiss-Peters) were used initially in selecting subjects, but not following treatment. Such information would have been useful in evaluating the generality of the treatment effects. This study is also limited in that no follow-up data are presented.

Gittelman-Klein et al. (1976) reported the use of a combined school and home behavior therapy program for hyperactive children between the ages of 6 and 12. The behaviors targeted in the classroom were such things as listening to the teacher, not calling out, not interrupting, not leaving seat, doing the work, and not disturbing others. Home behaviors included compliance, cooperation, and not fighting. For one group of children (N = 9), a placebo drug, contingency management in the classroom, and parent training were utilized over an 8-week period. Points could be earned in the classroom and later exchanged for reinforcement at home. A second group (N = 13) received behavior therapy as just described and stimulant medication, and a third group (N = 12) received methylphenidate alone. Drug dosage was increased throughout the study based on teacher and parent reports of problems. There was an average group daily dose of 35.6 mg. It is assumed that "placebo dose adjustments" were made in the behavior therapy–placebo condition as well, although this is nòt clear from the report. Although the authors indicate that rewards and punishments were revised as treatment progressed, it is not clear whether this involved "stronger rewards" if behavior did not change. The preprogram history of medication is also not clear from the report; i.e., were children in the behavior therapy–placebo condition taken off medication on entering the program?

After 8 weeks of treatment the interventions were evaluated using teacher ratings of hyperactivity, global ratings of overall improvement by teachers, mothers, and psychiatrists, and direct observations in the classroom. Although home behavior was being monitored as part of this ongoing study, it was not reported for this sample. The pattern of findings reported with respect to teacher ratings and classroom behavior showed significant beneficial effects for all treatments, with the methylphenidate–behavior therapy group showing the most improvement followed by the methylphenidate-alone group, and then the behavior therapy plus placebo group. The differences between the methylphenidate–behavior therapy and methylphenidate groups were negligible, whereas behavior therapy–placebo was less effective than methylphenidate alone on a number of measures. Similar trends were noted in the global improvement ratings by teachers and psychiatrists, although in no instance was there a significant difference between the methylphenidate-alone and behavior therapy groups on these measures. Mother ratings of improvement were generally positive and were not different across the groups.

This study by Gittelman-Klein et al. (1976) is noteworthy in its careful attention to design, selection of subjects, and use of observational measures for evaluating change. Although the authors are careful to point out the limitations of this study, the guarded, but nevertheless explicit, conclusions that they draw from their results are that medication is the most effective treatment of hyperactivity and that behavior therapy may be added if medication is not enough. The findings presented in this study must be considered in light of the facts that the subjects were "severely" disruptive and were treated with fairly large doses of stimulant medication, and the study was conducted over a short time period with no follow-up, does not include information regarding preintervention medication status, and provides no direct information about possible behavior changes in the home. In addition, it is not clear whether methylphenidate dosage was similar across the two drug conditions (this is not reported), nor is it clear whether the amount and quality of behavior therapy received was equivalent across the two groups receiving this treatment. For example, the number of contact hours with the therapists in each condition is not reported, nor is it evident that the therapist(s) were the same or different in the two behavioral treatment conditions. All of these factors create potentially serious problems in this study.

These comments are in no way intended to contradict the guarded conclusion of Gittelman-Klein et al. that medication is more effective than behavior therapy. Rather, they are presented to point out that trying to draw such conclusions makes little sense, since the question is too global. Medication is not a unitary treatment, and behavior therapy is even more diverse. Therefore, what is needed are empirical statements regarding the effectiveness and/or relative effectiveness of specific medication regimens, or specific behavior therapy interventions, for specific children, with specific behaviors in particular situations. Comparative studies like Gittelman-Klein et al. (1976) can contribute to the development of such empirical statements, although admittedly they are limited by their group design to discussions of average effects. On the other hand, such comparative therapy studies (Kiesler, 1971) have not provided singular conclusive statements that one brand of therapy is better than another, especially when applied to the treatment of an individual case—nor are they likely to in the future. It is unfortunate that Gittelman-Klein et al. (1976) interpreted their results in this fashion, since the empirical and methodological contribution of their study is enormous and is likely to be even greater when the rest of their findings are reported.

Douglas et al. (1976) employed counseling sessions with both teachers and parents in an intensive program of cognitive training with hyperactive children. Although the parents and teachers were counseled in and used contingency management on a limited but unspecified basis, the emphasis was on teaching parents and teachers the importance of helping the children to become self-controlling, self-monitoring, and self-reinforcing individuals. Contingency management was also employed on a limited basis in some of the cognitive training sessions. This is one of the few studies in which parents were trained in something other than contingency management. It is noteworthy as well in recognizing the important contribution of stimulus and reinforcement factors in the natural environment in the development and maintenance of self-controlling strategies. The effectiveness of the training program was assessed utilizing a number of cognitive, motor performance, and achievement measures, as well as teacher ratings. In general, the results favored the training group over no-treatment controls and some gains were maintained at a 3-month follow-up. Teacher ratings (CATRS) did not change as a function of treatment and because of practical difficulties no direct or parent-reported information was presented regarding behavior at home, although the description of subjects would suggest that problems at home were prevalent prior to intervention. It is difficult to evaluate the possible contribution of the family counseling sessions in this overall program since it included 24 hours of individual training with the child, six consultation sessions with the teacher, and 12 sessions with the parents (the length of these "consultation" sessions is not specified). The study does, however, point up the importance of involving family members and other agents as facilitators and reinforcers of self-controlling strategies.

ISSUES AND RECOMMENDATIONS

The studies described are representative of the types of behavioral interventions for the hyperactive child and his family that have been reported in the literature. These studies are few in number and, because of a number of methodological problems (O'Leary, 1977), are inconclusive with respect to assessing the potential benefit of behavioral interventions with hyperactive children. It is not that the data do not support this approach, but rather that the relevant studies have not yet been done. It is appropriate now to consider some of the limitations of previous studies and to make recommendations for future work in this area.

Small Number of Subjects

Despite the probable widespread clinical application of behavioral procedures with hyperactive children (Safer and Allen, 1976), *the numbers of subjects* involved in behavior therapy research studies have been relatively small (Cantwell, 1975). Although single-subject research is probably preferred for the evaluation of treatment effects (Hersen and Barlow, 1976), many of the studies have been case reports or anecdotal descriptions rather than systematically conducted, within-subject designs (e.g., multiple baseline, reversal, changing criterion). The relative paucity of good single-subject research with family intervention is likely related to the need for continuous performance measures in studies of this sort, combined with the difficulties and costs involved in obtaining such measures in the home.

Adequate Selection Criteria

It is likely that behavior therapists were initially more interested in demonstrating the general efficacy of behavioral procedures with disruptive children than they were in showing that these procedures were effective specifically with children labeled hyperactive. A consistent long-term clinical research program with hyperactive children paralleling those of Patterson and his colleagues (1976) with aggressive children and Lovaas and his colleagues (Lovaas et al., 1973) with autistic children did not appear early in the development of behavior therapy. In spite of its prevalence, an interest in behavioral interventions for hyperactivity was a relative latecomer in the child behavior therapy area. Although Patterson's early work (Patterson, 1965; Patterson et al., 1965) has been frequently cited as seminal in the behavioral treatment of hyperactivity, the focus of this research was as much with the effective demonstration of the behavioral techniques for problem behaviors as it was with the problem of hyperactivity per se.

The prevalence of "hyperactivity" and hyperactive behaviors across children and settings led to sometimes coincidental behavior therapy applications across a range of settings (hyperactive behaviors in the classroom, in the home, and in institutional settings) and populations (with retarded children, with severely brain-damaged children, and with autistic children). The general lack of attention to subject selection criteria that has been alluded to in criticisms of these studies is a problem only when the studies are used in support or refute of behavioral interventions with hyperactive children. However, it should be recognized that the main focus of many of these studies was not to demonstrate effectiveness with hyperactives. As behavior therapists become more interested in interventions specifically with hyperactives, and more generally with the problem of hyperactivity, it is likely that increasing attention will be given to adequate selection criteria, including direct observations with standardized code systems (Abikoff, Gittelman-Klein, and Klein, 1977; Williams and Vincent, 1977; Jacob, O'Leary, and Rosenblad, 1978), the use of standardized parent and teacher rating scales, standardized assessments of intellectual and cognitive functioning, and assessments of other subject characteristics, including the possibility of serious organic impairment, mental retardation, clinical history, etc. (Safer and Allen, 1976). A trend toward the use of more adequate selection criteria is already evident in some of the more recent behavioral studies. Berler and Romanczyk (1977) have recently described such a standardized selection battery as including intelligence measures (WISC-R, Peabody), achievement measures (Wide Range Achievement Test, Woodcock Reading Mastery Test), Bender-Gestalt Test, MFFT, Wepman Auditory Discrimination Test, rating scales (Conners Teacher, Werry-Weiss-Peters, Child Problem Behavior Checklist), physiological measures (heart rate, galvanic skin response) in response to various stimuli, Continuous Performance Test, physical and neurological examination, and in vivo observation.

Selection of Dependent Variables

As pointed out by O'Leary (1977) many of the dependent measures used in early studies were not *specific to hyperactivity*, nor were they measures that had been shown to be sensitive to drug treatments. Responses such as movement, on-task, looking, in-seat, aggression, noncompliance, and ritualistic behaviors were targeted for change, in addition to attentional measures. There is likely a need to develop and utilize dependent measures that reflect the attentional deficit characteristic of the disorder (Douglas, 1975). Kistner (1977) has recently recommended that multiple measures of attention be utilized, including behavioral observations, vigilance tasks, reaction-time tasks, and physiological measures. In general, there is a need to utilize multiple outcome measures in any treatment study with hyperactive children.

Since drug treatments are so prevalent, it is reasonable that behavioral interventions be evaluated utilizing some of the same measures that have been shown to be sensitive to drug treatments—specifically, standardized rating scales such as those developed by Conners and Werry, Weiss, and Peters. Several recent studies (O'Leary et al., 1976; Dubey et al., 1977a; Pelham, 1977) have utilized such measures, unfortunately at times in lieu of systematic observation by trained observers. It is equally reasonable to expect that drug studies, and especially behavior therapy–drug study comparisons, utilize measures that have been shown to be behavior therapy sensitive—particularly direct measures of observable behavior under naturalistic conditions. Several recent studies of drug effects (Cunningham and Barkley, 1978; Barkley and Cunningham, 1978a) and drug–behavior therapy comparisons (Gittelman-Klein et al., 1976) have included such measures.

Although behavioral studies with hyperactive children have frequently used direct observation measures in the classroom, in the laboratory (Seitz and Terdal, 1972), and less frequently in the home setting, the variations in the behaviors coded, as well as the definitions given to response topography represented by a given code, have been highly idiosyncratic to the particular study. So, for example, many different definitions may exist for attention or for distractibility. This lack of standardization parallels that found more generally for behavior therapy assessment (Mash and Terdal, 1976). The result is a confusing state of affairs in discussing or attempting to compare findings from different studies.

It is recommended that investigators using observational systems with hyperactive children first of all develop standard code systems that are sensitive to the problems of the hyperactive child *in the situation* for which the observation system is intended. Several code systems have recently been developed for observation of the hyperactive child in the classroom (Abikoff et al., 1977; Campbell et al., 1977; Williams and Vincent, 1977; Jacob et al., 1978). These code systems have shown some reliability and validity. In comparing the Abikoff et al. (1977) and Jacob et al. (1978) code systems with the Williams and Vincent (1977) code system, the former focus entirely on negative behaviors, whereas the latter includes several positive categories as well. In addition, both the Campbell et al. (1977) and Williams and Vincent (1977) codes are sequential and look at the teacher and peer response to the hyperactive child, whereas the Abikoff et al. (1977) code looks at the behavior of the child in isolation and is therefore somewhat restricted in its potential for generating an adequate functional analysis or for assessing social system changes. Unfortunately, although these codes are sensitive to the hyperactive child's classroom behavior and were standardized with hyperactive children, there is little cross-code standardization. So, for example, even with a simple motor response like "standing" the definitions are different in two of the code systems. It would be desirable that standard definitions be used. By doing so, investigators interested in utilizing only one or two specific behavioral codes could draw on the standard definition in the more general code system. An appeal for such standardization of measures has been made for research in the general area of child development (Bell and Hertz, 1976).

There exists the same need for standardized observational measures in the home and laboratory. There have been no systems devised specifically for observation of the hyperactive child in the home setting. There are, however, several standard codes that have been used generally for observation of problem children in the home setting (Patterson et al., 1969; Bernal and North, 1972; Mash, Terdal, and Anderson, 1973; Mash and McElwee, 1976; Wahler, House, and Stambaugh, 1976). All of these codes have categories relevant to the behavior of hyperactive children and their families in the home and could be adapted to meet the assessment needs characterizing this population.

The dependent measures used in behavioral studies have too infrequently assessed the social and environmental events surrounding the occurrence of hyperactive behavior. With few exceptions (e.g., Campbell, 1975; Campbell et al., 1977; Humphries, Kinsbourne, and Swanson, 1978; Jacob et al., 1978) most studies have looked only at the behavior of the hyperactive child independent of situational context. Although broad situational characteristics such as home versus classroom or structured versus nonstructured activities provide some information, they are not likely to reveal the specific controlling and maintaining events for hyperactivity. What is needed here is a careful description of the *immediate* context for behavior. Such information can be utilized in the design of behavioral interventions, and also creates the possibility of identifying whether or not changes as a function of treatment are related to specific changes in the behavior of social agents, i.e., teachers and parents. To date, few studies evaluating behavior therapy with hyperactive children have utilized parent-child, teacher-child, child-peer, or child-sibling interactions as the dependent measure. It should be noted that many of the so-called secondary symptoms of hyperactivity are social in nature, e.g., aggressive interpersonal behavior, and have been related to varying parent styles (Paternite, Loney, and Langhorne, 1976). On the other hand, "primary symptoms," e.g., hyperactivity, inattention, and fidgetiness, were not as well predicted by parenting styles (Paternite et al., 1976). These findings, although interesting and suggestive, have utilized global measures of parental style. More direct measures of parenting behavior as it affects, and is affected by, hyperactive behavior will likely promote better understanding of the relationship between the variables. Hopefully, such studies will help us to better understand the home environment of the hyperactive child.

Confounding of Treatments

Werry (1968) states that, since the hyperactive child is frequently multiply handicapped, a single remediation approach is not likely to be sufficient. Several authors have concurred in advocating multimodal treatments of the hyperactive child (Feighner and Feighner, 1974; Ross and Ross, 1976; Safer and Allen, 1976). Such multiple treatment approaches are viewed as enhancing the probability of clinical success; however, when applied in an unsystematic fashion multiple treatments make it difficult to identify the active ingredients in therapy.

Most behavior therapy interventions have involved the simultaneous use of multiple approaches, including reinforcement, modeling, token systems, punishment, videotape feedback, behavior recording, etc. Parametric studies are needed to assess the individual and interacting effects associated with varying treatments. One might argue that such studies are impractical in the number of groups required to compare various procedures, and unethical since they require witholding potentially effective treatments from particular groups of children. However, as Hersen and Barlow (1976) point out, single-subject designs, particularly those using multiple baselines, are uniquely suited to such comparative and parametric study. Such designs do not require large numbers of subjects, nor do they require witholding treatment for long time periods.

Behavior therapy interventions are often confounded in failing to take into account the medication status and drug dosage of the child. Behavioral interventions while a child is on medication cannot, without adequate design (e.g., Gittelman-Klein et al., 1976), assess the independent and interacting effects of the two treatments. On the other hand, withdrawing medication at the time that a behavioral program is instituted may present a particularly disruptive and unrepresentative baseline. As demonstrated by Sulzbacher and his co-workers (Sulzbacher, 1973, 1975; Strong, Sulzbacher, and Kirkpatrick, 1974; Shafto and Sulzbacher, 1977) and others (Cunningham and Barkley, 1978; Wulbert and Dries, 1977), single-subject designs are well suited to studies examining drug-behavior relationships in treatment.

Setting Generality

In addition to the use of many treatments simultaneously, behavior therapy has also been conducted simultaneously in several settings, i.e., school, home, and clinic. It is not uncommon, however, for behavior to be monitored in only one of these situations (Douglas et al., 1976). The multiple baseline design seems most applicable for behavior therapy studies that successively introduce treatments across settings. Such a multiple baseline strategy was used in a study by Wulbert and Dries (1977) to assess the generalization of a clinic treatment to the home setting. Unfortunately, the results of this study are confounded by the simultaneous rather than successive introduction of treatments in the clinic and home.

Simultaneous monitoring of behaviors across various settings is sorely needed for a number of reasons. First of all, it is important to assess the generality of effects associated with varying treatments. For example, would a self-control program be more likely to produce generalized effects as compared with a reinforcement program in the classroom where the discriminative cues for responding are closely related to the situation? Few behavior therapy studies with hyperactive children have attempted to assess the effects of the program in nontreated settings. Some studies have found no generalization to the school situation following treatment in the home (Wahler, 1975; Johnson, Bolstad, and Lobitz, 1976). As well as no effect, it is also possible that positive behavior changes in one setting may be correlated with opposite effects in a nontreated situation. Johnson et al. (1976) and Wahler (1975) have noted such "negative contrast effects" in their treatment of problem children, i.e., as things improved at home, they got worse at school.

Secondly, simultaneous monitoring of behavior across settings permits the examination of intra- and interbehavior covariations. Some behaviors may show high cross-situational correlations, whereas others may be quite situation specific. It has been reported, for example (Mischel, 1973; Wahler et al., 1977; Mash and Mercer, 1979), that deviant children tend to show greater cross-situational consistency, suggesting that they do not regulate their behavior in relation to situational demands. This deficiency has been noted in hyperactive children under laboratory conditions. It would be interesting to see if these relationships hold up under more naturalistic circumstances. Rapoport and Benoit (1975) have reported some degree of consistency in the behavior of hyperactives across the clinic and home settings.

The relationship between different responses both within and across settings has some important implications with regard to functional response classes. If, for example, low rates of independent toy play in the home are highly correlated with disruptive behavior at bedtime, it may be possible to reduce disruptiveness at bedtime by increasing independent toy play. Such interventions have been reported (Wahler et al., 1977) and the potential use of functional response classes in the design of behavioral intervention strategies for hyperactive children is enormous.

Parent Training

Several detailed therapist manuals describing varying formats for training parents in behavior modification skills are currently available (Miller, 1975; Patterson et al., 1975). In addition, a number of reviews (Berkowitz and Graziano, 1972; Johnson and Katz, 1973; O'Dell, 1974; Mash, Hamerlynck, and Handy, 1976; Mash, Handy, and Hamerlynck, 1976; Reisinger, Ora, and Frangia, 1976; Graziano, 1977) have documented the efficacy of such parent training programs in producing at least short-term changes in child behavior. Although several writers (Simmons, 1975; Willis and Lovaas, 1977) have outlined the general strategy for training parents of hyperactive children, there have been few systematic studies investigating parent training efforts with this population. It should be noted that, both with respect to the guidelines that have been set forth and in relation to the few studies that have been carried out, the interventions are not tailored to, nor are they specific to, the problems of the hyperactive child. The approach is one of teaching good contingency management "in general," which might then be applied to any behavior of interest.

It is likely that there will be an increase in the conduct and systematic evaluation of courses for parents of hyperactive children. Such work should proceed with full recognition of some of the limitations that currently exist in evaluating the effects of behavioral parent training programs in general.

In spite of the increasing use and marked success of parenting programs in achieving short-term changes, a number of prevalent issues still remain.

1. The generality of effects for family interventions has been questioned. It is unclear that changes endure over time, generalize across settings, or affect nontreated behaviors or family members (Forehand and Atkeson, 1977). In part, this state of affairs is related to the use of subjective and biased measures for evaluating change rather than a reliance on independent observers.
2. There is little knowledge regarding the specific components of behavioral interventions that may be producing change. Behavioral programs for parents have included a range of potentially therapeutic ingredients, including instruction, feedback, role playing, and model-

ing, and it is only speculation as to which of these ingredients are necessary conditions in producing change.

3. We have no real knowledge base as to why behavioral interventions with families are effective. That is, the process leading to change is ill-understood. The assumption is, for example, that parents who are instructed in behavioral procedures will apply such procedures and it is this alteration in parental consequence style that is responsible for change. This is purely assumptive in that this is most often not monitored and therefore we do not know whether the changes are occurring for the purported reasons. It is equally plausible that correlated variables (e.g., parental attitude, time spent with child) may be the common factors in producing therapeutic change.

4. Behavioral interventions with families have, for the most part, not looked at the entire social system in which the child operates. Parent training has been the rule, and, although some of the major behavioral efforts in this area have used combined home and school programs (e.g., those of Patterson, Bernal, Wahler, and O'Leary), each has had a particular emphasis and, as major research efforts, these programs are not representative of many other applications that have been reported.

5. Behavioral interventions with families have not addressed themselves to parental attitudes in determinations of deviancy, in spite of the fact that such attitudes seem to serve as a focal point in the family unit and also determine whether or not the child is referred for treatment.

6. The natural mediator assumption put forth by Tharp and Wetzel (1969) has been such a powerful force in determining the nature of family interventions (parent training) that the possibilities for other more powerful interventions have not been explored. The natural mediator hypothesis has been powerful in a number of ways—conceptually, in relation to generality, and in relation to efficiency. However, it has not been tested. That is, it is possible that direct intervention with children related to home problem situations by trained professionals may be more powerful and enduring than mediated family behavior therapy. It is also possible that parents may be utilized in treatment in more diverse ways. For the most part, parents in behavioral intervention programs have served as contingency managers for their children's disruptive behaviors in the home (Pelham, 1976) and/or as back-up reinforcing agents for appropriate classroom behaviors (O'Leary et al., 1976). It is possible that parents could be involved in other ways, for example, as cueing,

modeling, and reinforcing agents in helping hyperactive children to develop more effective self-controlling strategies (Douglas et al., 1976). Some studies have also shown that under certain circumstances parents may be effective remediation specialists for academic behaviors (Ryback and Staats, 1970; Skindrud, 1972).

7. Since it is not clear that parents of nonproblem children are effective contingency managers, training parents in behavior modification skills may not be sufficient as a treatment goal (Forehand and Wells, 1977).

These are some of the current status issues in behavior therapy with families. It is within this overall context that behavioral parent interventions for children exhibiting hyperactive behavior must be considered.

Follow-up

There is little currently available information regarding the long-term effects of behavior therapy programs for hyperactive children (Brundage-Aguar et al., 1977; O'Leary, 1977). This state of affairs is not unique to behavioral management with hyperactive children, but characterizes the field of behavior therapy as a whole (Atthowe, 1973; Keely, Shemberg, and Carbonell, 1976; Forehand, and Atkeson, 1977). The problem is also not unique to behavior therapy, since the long-term effects of drug treatments are also not known.

Most of the behavioral treatments with hyperactive children have thus far failed to provide any information beyond the termination of treatment. Where follow-up information is provided, it is usually for a short time period or based on highly subjective or anecdotal material, obtained, for example, in a brief telephone contact. Typically, the rationale for selecting particular follow-up intervals is not made clear and there have been no guidelines for designating the length of follow-up intervals in relation to specific characteristics of the behavior or situation under study. For example, one might speculate that a behavioral program designed to alter inattention might require longer follow-up than one that alters excessive activity in a young child (Mash, 1976; Hartmann, Roper, and Gelfand, 1977).

Although there has been a general consensus that follow-up studies should be done, the practicalities, methodological difficulties, and costs associated with such longitudinal studies contribute to their infrequency. Subject attrition rates are typically high. For example, in one longitudinal study of hyperactive children (Campbell et al., 1977) over 40% of the original sample could not be located at follow-up, and high numbers of treatment drop-outs are also not infrequent, even over short time intervals (Dubey, Kaufman, and O'Leary, 1977b). Mash and Terdal (1977, 1978) have recently presented guidelines for the conduct of adequate follow-up studies in behavior therapy.

It is likely that hyperactivity is frequently a chronic rather than an acute condition, and consequently the need for on-going follow-up assessment is especially evident. In conducting follow-up studies with hyperactive children, investigators should be sensitive to some of the varying purposes. In addition to those follow-up studies that are exclusively evaluative and attempt to assess the long-term outcomes of treatment, ongoing diagnostic follow-ups that attempt to determine if further intervention is required, and, if so, what type, are also extremely important. Follow-up assessments that include measures of both behavior and situational context are likely to provide the most useful types of diagnostic information.

Individual and Situational Differences

The increasing recognition that hyperactivity is not a unitary phenomenon (Marwit and Stenner, 1972; Ney, 1974) has led to a greater interest in identifying those child, family, or situational characteristics that may be associated with varying treatment outcomes, or would predict a relative advantage of one form of treatment over another. Barkley (1976) has reviewed some of the factors that might be involved in predicting the response of hyperkinetic children to stimulant drug treatment. Similar information is needed in relation to response to varying behavioral interventions with hyperactive children.

Severity of the Problem

Most interventions have shown little consideration for the initial baseline severity of the problem. This characteristic has not been taken into account, and the therapeutic programs prescribed tend to be similar regardless of the degree of hyperactivity exhibited, which is frequently not assessed. It is likely that more severe problems would require both qualitatively and quantitatively different interventions and that initial severity might predict compliance with, or outcome for, the therapeutic procedures. For example, Dubey et al. (1977b) report that the initial Werry-Weiss-Peters scores of children whose parents dropped out of their training program were higher than those who stayed.

Central Nervous System Arousal

The hyperactive child's pretreatment level of CNS arousal may be a factor predicting differential responsiveness to treatment, although the available data in this area are presently minimal. A review of psychophysiological findings with hyperactive children by Hastings and Barkley (1978) suggests that some subgroups of hyperactive children may be underarousable and consequently less reactive to certain types of environmental stimulation. If this observation is confirmed in future research, then there would be clear implications for behavioral interventions that were based on the rearrangement of environmental antecedents and consequents. More research is needed in this area.

Attributional System of the Child

Whalen and Henker (1976) and Bugental, Whalen, and Henker (1977) have considered the causal attribution system of the hyperactive child as a potentially important subject variable in predicting response to treatment. Bugental et al. (1977) carried out a 2-month classroom tutoring program in which medicated or nonmedicated (no drug or dosage information is given) 7–12-year-old hyperactive boys were exposed to self-control training or social reinforcement for task attention. Each child's view of personal causality (PC) for *school success and failure* was also assessed, and groups were formed based on attribution-intervention congruence. Congruent groups were high PC children in the self-control condition and low PC children in the social reinforcement condition. Incongruent groups were high PC in the social reinforcement condition and low PC in the self-control condition. It was found that children in the congruent groups showed a significantly greater reduction in Porteus Maze qualitative errors than those in the noncongruent conditions. For the same Porteus Maze measure, social reinforcement procedures were significantly more effective for the medicated children, whereas self-control procedures were slightly more effective for the nonmedicated children but not significantly so. Teacher ratings were unaffected by any of the treatments. Although this study is important in pointing out the possibility of treatment-subject interactions, it would be premature to draw any specific conclusions regarding the relationship between locus of causality and type of treatment. The study considered only one area of personal causality (school success or failure), looked at short-term changes on a single measure, and showed no effects of treatment on teacher ratings. It is also possible that the medicated and nonmedicated groups were not equivalent, since teacher ratings, which have been shown to be sensitive to drug effects, did not differ for the two groups. Research is needed to further assess the role of attributional systems in the design of intervention programs.

Self-Esteem

If hyperactive children are likely to exhibit a lower level of self-esteem, as some have suggested (Loney et al., 1976; Campbell et al., 1977) specific interventions might be designed to take this into account.

Some studies have attempted to enhance the child's self-concept through the use of self-modeling procedures in which the child is given videotape feedback of himself performing successfully. Videotapes of successful performance are constructed either by editing out inappropriate sequences or turning off the camera when the child is distracted or disruptive (Bugental et al., 1977). Such procedures are interesting but require further investigation. If self-modeling is to be used in attempting to enhance self-esteem or self-concept, consideration should be given to the literature demonstrating the relative effectiveness of coping models (Kazdin, 1973). Feedback that shows the child "gaining control" over responding is likely to be more effective than feedback involving only successful performance. In any case, the design of behavioral intervention programs has not been sensitive to initial differences in the child's self-esteem and the possible relationship of this to treatment outcome.

Response to Reinforcement

The laboratory studies cited earlier *suggest* that hyperactive children may respond uniquely to reinforcement and punishment (Douglas, 1975). The proposed unique response pattern should be considered in developing behavior programs. The response to varying reinforcement conditions may be unique not only to hyperactive children as a group, but also to individual children within that group. Consequently, the need for a careful analysis and identification of potentially reinforcing events is important. The methods for conducting such reinforcer assessments include surveys (Clement and Richard, 1976), observation (Bersoff and Moyer, 1976), structured interviews (Holland, 1970), and empirical tests (Fagot and Patterson, 1969), and have been described in detail elsewhere (Mash and Terdal, 1976). It would seem more fruitful to account for individual differences in response to reinforcement through such assessments rather than to generate laboratory-produced generalizations regarding the manner in which hyperactive children as a group respond to reinforcement.

Parenting Style and Socioeconomic Status

Some studies have found that parenting style and/or socioeconomic status (SES) were correlated with a positive response to medication

(Loney et al., 1975), whereas others have found no evidence for the claim (Loney et al., 1976). The role of these variables in the design and choice of behavior therapy programs is also important. For example, previous research has suggested that the educational level of parents may predict outcomes in behavioral parenting programs (Anchor and Thomason, 1977).

Paternite et al. (1976) have shown that the "primary symptoms" of hyperactivity (e.g., inattention) are less related to SES and parenting styles (e.g., love-hostility, autonomy-control) than are secondary symptoms such as aggressiveness and self-esteem. To the extent that such relationships may be predictive of parent responses as controlling variables, it is possible that behavioral programs with parents might focus more on some of these secondary symptoms, whereas alternative interventions (e.g., biofeedback, cognitive training, or medication) might be used in overcoming some of the attentional deficits.

Parental Attitudes and Norms

In considering the label of hyperactivity, it is evident that the designation is based on social labeling factors. Several writers have implicated parental norms as being important in determining whether or not a child is viewed as hyperactive (Conrad, 1976; Ross, 1976). It is also the case that such norms may persist despite objective changes in child behavior (Patterson et al., 1975) or shift without concomitant changes in child behavior. For example, Barkley and Cunningham (1978a) noted that, although hyperactive children were not more socially responsive while on medication, their mothers tended to perceive their behavior as more acceptable. Therefore, in considering the design and outcome evaluation of behavioral interventions, some measures of parental norms for the appropriateness of various child behaviors in particular situations would be useful. For example, do parents of hyperactive children tend to have more or less tolerance for particular child behaviors, and to what extent do these norms relate to how the parents responds to their child? We have recently attempted to measure such norms through the utilization of standard behavior-situation matrices (Figure 1), in which parents of hyperactive and nonhyperactive children are asked to rate the perceived appropriateness of various child behaviors in particular situations. This work is still in a preliminary stage; however, possible differences in norms between parents of hyperactive and nonhyperactive children and in the extent to which within-group normative differences might relate to parental reactions to the child should contribute valuable information to the design of different intervention programs.

Scoring

1 = The behavior is extremely inappropriate
in this situation.
9 = The behavior is extremely appropriate
in this situation.

Sample Items

1. Daydream while watching TV.
2. Cry in the car.
3. Run in the supermarket.
4. Laugh in the classroom.

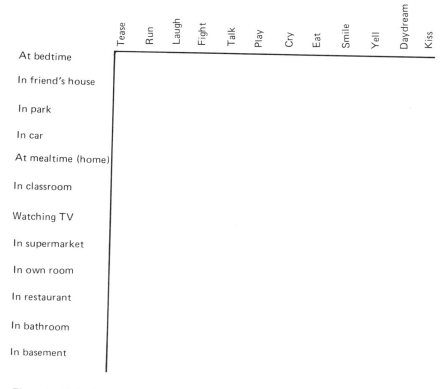

Figure 1.   Behavior-situation matrix.

Environmental Structure

Some studies have shown a relationship between environmental structure and the effects of medication. For example, it has been suggested that medication may be effective in architecturally open classrooms but might have the opposite effect in formal classroom arrangements (O'Leary, 1977). Jacob et al. (1978) reported that hyperactive children had significantly higher levels of hyperactivity than control children in a formal classroom setting, but reported no differences in a more informal, or "open," setting. Similar factors might also mediate the effectiveness of various behavioral intervention programs, e.g., token economy versus social attention, and should be carefully assessed as part of the initial functional analysis. Several studies have also shown that changes in the physical structure or organization of settings can have dramatic effects on behavior, and such stimulus control programs offer reasonable alternatives to those based exclusively on contingency management (Risley, 1977).

Lack of a Social System Emphasis

In spite of the behavioral view of hyperactivity as a situation-related problem, behavioral investigators have taken a narrow approach in their studies with hyperactive children. Frequently the functional analyses are incomplete because they do not include home or school information, and there is currently a minimal amount of direct observational information available that describes the interactions between hyperactive children and their parents, teachers, peers, and siblings. This is true despite the fact that the problem is heavily embedded in this social context. It is encouraging to see the emergence of studies that have attempted to observe such interactions directly (Campbell, 1973; Campbell et al., 1977; Cunningham and Barkley, 1978; Barkley and Cunningham, 1978a), and more are needed.

The treatment targets of many programs of behavioral intervention have frequently looked only at the child. Changes in other aspects of the child's social system as a function of treatment have not been examined. Little attention has been given to the effect of the hyperactive child in his social system, despite the fact that we have long recognized the reciprocal nature of child-environment relationships (Bell and Harper, 1977). Campbell et al. (1977), for example, report that teachers tend to be more negative toward nonhyperactive children when a hyperactive-disruptive child is in the class. Williams and Vincent (1977) report similar findings. Arnold et al. (1975) and Mash and Mercer (1979) report high rates of problems in siblings of problem children, and siblings of hyperactives have been shown to be more frequently hyperactive than siblings of nonhyperactive children. It is interesting to note that, although teachers may respond more negatively to the hyperactive child (Williams and Vincent, 1977), mothers may actually be more encouraging (Campbell, 1973). Consequently, the child may be receiving inconsistent feedback for the same behaviors.

Lack of an Adequate Conceptual Model

Behavioral effects in the study and treatment of hyperactive children and their families have not been guided by a well-formulated conceptual model. Consequently, much of the research is fragmented and frequently the interventions that are carried out do not follow from careful functional analysis, i.e., they are not based on predicted or empirically demonstrated factors that may be contributing to the maintenance of hyperactivity. Many treatment programs are used because they have been successful with other kinds of problems and their content does not reflect procedures specific to what we know about the hyperactive child and his family.

In an intensive research-clinical program over a span of 10 years, Patterson (1976) has formulated a developmental model for aggressive behavior in children that identifies some of the social variables that maintain the behavior and the effect of such behaviors on the family system. Aggression is viewed as a class of coercive behaviors that is maintained by negative reinforcement. The reciprocal nature of the parent-child and child-sibling relationship is given emphasis and the manner in which the aggressive child may promote nonadaptive behaviors in other family members is considered. Interestingly, despite the relevance of this model, and the potential for understanding hyperactive children and their families, with few exceptions (Barkley and Cunningham, 1978c) this work goes virtually uncited in the literature on hyperactivity. References to Patterson's work in the hyperactivity literature typically are to early studies (Patterson, 1965; Patterson et al., 1965) that do not reflect the massive research program that followed, despite the fact that there is considerable overlap in the two populations, i.e., hyperactive children are frequently socially aggressive, and difficulties in school are prevalent for both populations. In fact, many of the aggressive children Patterson has worked with were previously diagnosed as hyperactive. The conceptual model, treatment procedures, and methodology developed by Patterson should be tested out in populations of hyperactive children. This should serve to give some focus to research and intervention in this area.

Another well-developed model for examining child deviancy has been described by Wahler et al. (1977). This model provides social systems emphasis to the study of the child and attempts to identify covariations in behaviors for individual children and across settings. A consideration of this approach also seems fruitful in providing a conceptual base for the behavioral study of hyperactive children.

Need for Early Intervention

Much of the behavior therapy demonstrations have been carried out with school-age children, since it is in this situation where the problem is more likely to manifest itself (Ross and Ross, 1976). However, as several writers have noted, mothers frequently report more difficult behavior from infancy (Campbell et al., 1976; Ross and Ross, 1976). Campbell et al. (1977) have shown a relationship between nursery school behavior and later classroom responding, suggesting that hyperactivity may be identified at earlier ages. Newborn minor physical anomalies have also been shown to predict problems at later ages (Waldrop et al., 1978). It is with such early identification and intervention that behavioral programs would seem to hold special promise. Procedures are needed for early identification so that anticipatory parental guidance and early teacher consultation may be carried out (Schrager and Lindy, 1970). A major test for behavior therapy effectiveness with hyperactives would be one in which a preschool home-clinic intervention could reduce or circumvent the social, behavioral, and academic difficulties that might be predicted to occur. Such a preventative approach is sorely needed.

Cost-Benefit Analyses

Many writers in the behavior therapy area have noted the importance of considering the costs associated with behavioral interventions relative to alternative treatments (Davidson, Clark, and Hamerlynck, 1974; Patterson et al., 1975). Such consideration seems especially relevant in the treatment of hyperactive children. The efficacy of stimulant drugs for short-term behavioral management, their ease of use as compared to the time and expense involved in parent training efforts (O'Leary and Pelham, 1978), the urgency of many parent and teacher requests for immediate action, and the fact that a large proportion of hyperactive children come from lower socioeconomic groups are all factors that must be considered in relation to the extent to which behavioral procedures will find extensive use in the treatment of hyperactive children and their families. There is no question that behavioral interventions cost more than drug treatments. It remains to be seen whether their benefits in terms of early intervention and remediation of academic and social difficulties outweigh the additional costs. It is therefore important that behavioral investigators give careful attention to the development of programs for hyperactive children that are not only effective but also economically viable.

CONCLUSIONS

A review of behavioral interventions for hyperactive children and their families shows that a wide range of procedures have been utilized for a diverse range of problems. Recent work has shown an increasing concern for the use of adequate selection criteria, multiple outcome measures and longer follow-up intervals. More empirical information is needed before the effectiveness of specific behavioral interventions can be evaluated; however, it is unlikely that global questions such as "Is behavior therapy effective?" or "Is behavior therapy more effective than drug treatment?" can ever be answered. It is recommended that future behavioral investigations proceed from a more adequate conceptual framework, with a greater focus on the hyperactive child as a member of a larger interacting social system, and adopt a more preventative approach emphasizing early intervention.

ACKNOWLEDGMENT

The authors would like to thank Russell Barkley for his helpful comments. During the preparation of this chapter, Dr. Mash was supported by a Canadian council leave fellowship and Mr. Dalby by a Canadian Council Doctoral Fellowship.

REFERENCES

Abikoff, H., Gittelman-Klein, R., and Klein, D. F. 1977. Validation of a classroom observation code for hyperactive children. J. Consult. Clin. Psychol. 45:772–783.

Alabiso, F. 1975. Operant control of attention behavior: A treatment for hyperactivity. Behav. Ther. 6:39–42.

Allen, R. P. 1977. Drug treatment of hyperactivity. Paper presented at the meeting of the Association for the Advancement of Behavior Therapy, December, Atlanta, Georgia.

Allen, K. E., Henke, L. B., Harris, F. R., Baer, D. M., and Reynolds, N. J. 1967. Control of hyperactivity by social reinforcement of attending behavior. J. Educ. Psychol. 58:231–237.

Anchor, K. N., and Thomason, T. C. 1977. A comparison of two parent-training models with educated parents. J. Community Psychol. 5:134–141.

Arnold, J. E., Levine, A. G., and Patterson, G. R. 1975. Change in sibling behavior following family intervention. J. Consult. Clin. Psychol. 43:683–688.

Atthowe, J. M. 1973. Behavior innovation and persistence. Am. Psychol. 28:34–41.

Ayllon, T., Garber, S., and Pisor, K. 1975. The elimination of discipline problems through a combined school-home motivational system. Behav. Ther. 6:616–626.

Ayllon, T., Layman, D., and Burke, S. 1972. Disruptive behavior and reinforcement of academic performance. Psychol. Record 22:315–323.

Ayllon, T., Layman, D., and Kandel, H. J. 1975. A behavioral-educational alternative to drug control of hyperactive children. J. Appl. Behav. Anal. 8:137–146.

Ayllon, T., and Roberts, M. 1974. Eliminating discipline problems by strengthening academic performance. J. Appl. Behav. Anal. 7:71–76.

Ayllon, T., and Rosenbaum, M. S. 1977. The behavioral treatment of disruption and hyperactivity in school settings. In B. B. Lahey and A. E. Kazdin (eds.), Advances in Clinical Child Psychology, Vol. 1, pp. 85–118. Plenum Publishing Corp., New York.

Bachrach, A. J., and Quigley, W. A. 1966. Direct methods of treatment. In I. A. Berg and L. A. Pennington (eds.), Introduction to Clinical Psychology, 3d ed., pp. 482–560. Ronald Press, New York.

Bailey, J. S., Wolf, M. M., and Phillips, E. L. 1970. Home-based reinforcement and the modification of pre-delinquents' classroom behavior. J. Appl. Behav. Anal. 3:223–233.

Bandura, A. 1977. Social Learning Theory. Prentice-Hall, Inc., Englewood Cliffs, N.J.

Barkley, R. A. 1976. Predicting the response of hyperkinetic children to stimulant drugs: A review. J. Abnorm. Child Psychol. 4:327–348.

Barkley, R. A. 1977. A review of stimulant drug research with hyperactive children. J. Child Psychol. Psychiatry 18:137–165.

Barkley, R. A., Copeland, A. P., and Sivage, C. 1978. A self-control classroom for hyperactive and impulsive children. Unpublished manuscript, University of Oregon Health Sciences Center.

Barkley, R. A., and Cunningham, C. E. 1978a. The effects of Ritalin on the mother-child interactions of hyperactive children. Arch. Gen. Psychiatry. In press.

Barkley, R. A., and Cunningham, C. E. 1978b. Do stimulant drugs improve the academic performance of hyperkinetic children? A review of outcome studies. Clin. Pediatr. 17:85–92.

Barkley, R. A., and Cunningham, C. E. 1978c. Stimulant drugs and the social interactions of hyperactive children. Unpublished manuscript, Medical College of Wisconsin.

Bell, R. Q., and Harper, L. V. 1977. Child Effects on Adults. Lawrence Erlbaum Associates, Hillsdale, N.J.

Bell, R. Q., and Hertz, T. W. 1976. Toward more comparability and generalizability of developmental research. Child Dev. 47:6–13.

Bender, N. N. 1976. Self-verbalization versus tutor verbalization in modifying impulsivity. J. Educ. Psychol. 68:347–354.

Berkowitz, B. P., and Graziano, A. M. 1972. Training parents as behavior therapists: A review. Behav. Res. Ther. 10:297–317.

Berler, E. S., and Romanczyk, R. G. 1977. Assessment of the learning disabled and hyperactive child: Therapeutic and research issues. Paper presented at the meeting of the Association for the Advancement of Behavior Therapy, December, Atlanta, Georgia.

Bernal, M. E., and North, J. A. 1972. A system for scoring home and school behaviors. Unpublished manuscript, University of Denver.

Bersoff, D. N., and Moyer, D. 1976. Positive reinforcement observation schedule (PROS): Development and use. In E. J. Mash and L. G. Terdal (eds.), Behavior Therapy Assessment: Diagnosis, Design and Evaluation, pp. 241–257. Springer, New York.

Black, A. H., and Cott, A. 1977. A perspective on biofeedback. In J. Beatty and H. Legewie (eds.), Biofeedback and Behavior, pp. 7–19. Plenum Publishing Corp., New York.

Bornstein, P. H., and Quevillon, R. P. 1976. The effects of a self-instructional package on overactive preschool boys. J. Appl. Behav. Anal. 9:179–188.

Braud, L. W. 1975. The effects of EMG biofeedback and progressive relaxation upon hyperactivity and its behavioral concomitants. Paper presented at the meeting of the Biofeedback Research Society, Colorado Springs, Colorado.

Braud, L. W., Lupin, M. N., and Braud, W. G. 1975. The use of electromyographic biofeedback in the control of hyperactivity. J. Learn. Disabil. 8:420–425.

Brundage-Aguar, D., Forehand, R., and Ciminero, A. R. 1977. A review of treatment approaches for hyperactive behavior. J. Clin. Child Psychol. 3:3–10.

Bryant, D. M., and Hunter, S. H. 1977. Is biofeedback training really beneficial for attention-problem children? Paper presented at the meeting of the Association for the Advancement of Behavior Therapy, December, Atlanta, Georgia.

Bugental, D. B., Whalen, C. K., and Henker, B. 1977. Causal attributions of hyperactive children and motivational assumptions of two behavior-change approaches: Evidence for an interactionist position. Child Dev. 48:874–884.

Burns, B. J. 1972. The effect of self-directed verbal commands on arithmetic performance and activity level of urban hyperactive children. (Doctoral dissertation, Boston College, 1972.) Dissertation Abstracts International 33:1782B (Microfilm No. 72–22, 884).

Camp, B. W., Blom, G. E., Herbert, F., and van Doorninck, W. J. 1977. "Think aloud": A program for developing self-control in young aggressive boys. J. Abnorm. Child Psychol. 5:157–169.

Campbell, S. B. 1973. Mother-child interaction in reflective, impulsive and hyperactive children. Dev. Psychol. 8:341–349.

Campbell, S. B. 1975. Mother-child interaction: A comparison of hyperactive, learning disabled and normal boys. Am. J. Orthopsychiatry 45:51–57.

Campbell, S. B., Endman, M. W., and Bernfeld, G. 1977. A three-year follow-up of hyperactive preschoolers in elementary school. J. Child Psychol. Psychiatry 18:239–249.

Cantwell, D. P. 1975. A critical review of therapeutic modalities with hyperactive children. In D. P. Cantwell (ed.), The Hyperactive Child: Diagnosis, Management, Current Research, pp. 173–189. Halsted Press, New York.

Christensen, D. E. 1975. Effects of combining methylphenidate and a classroom token system in modifying hyperactive behavior. Am. J. Ment. Defic. 80:266–276.

Christensen, D. E., and Sprague, R. L. 1973. Reduction of hyperactive behavior by conditioning procedures alone and combined with methylphenidate (Ritalin). Behav. Res. Ther. 11:331–334.

Clement, P. W., and Richard, R. C. 1976. Identifying reinforcers for children: A children's reinforcement survey. In E. J. Mash and L. G. Terdal (eds.), Behavior Therapy Assessment: Diagnosis, Design and Evaluation, pp. 207–216. Springer, New York.

Cohen, N. 1970. Physiological concomitants of attention in hyperactive children. Diss. Abstr. Int. 32:553B.

Colpaert, F. C. 1977. Drug-produced cues and states: Some theoretical and methodological inferences. In H. Lal (ed.), Discriminative Stimulus Properties of Drugs, pp. 5–20. Plenum Publishing Corp., New York.

Conrad, P. 1976. Identifying Hyperactive Children. D..C. Heath, Toronto.

Conrad, W., and Insel, J. 1967. Anticipating the response to amphetamine therapy in the treatment of hyperkinetic children. Pediatrics 40:96–98.

Craighead, W. E., Kazdin, A. E., and Mahoney, M. J. 1976. Behavior Modification: Principles, Issues and Applications. Houghton Mifflin Company, Boston.

Cunningham, C. E., and Barkley, R. A. 1978. The effects of Ritalin on the mother-child interactions of hyperactive identical twins. Dev. Med. Child Neurol. 20:634–642.

Dalby, J. T., Kinsbourne, M., Swanson, J. M., and Sobol, M. P. 1977. Hyperactive children's underuse of learning time: Correction by stimulant treatment. Child Dev. 48:1448–1453.

Davidson, P. O., Clark, F. W., and Hamerlynck, L. A. 1974. Evaluation of Behavior Programs in Community, Residential and School Settings. Research Press, Champaign, Ill.

Doubros, S. G., and Daniels, G. J. 1966. An experimental approach to the reduction of overactive behavior. Behav. Res. Ther. 4:251–258.

Douglas, V. 1972. Stop, look, and listen: The problem of sustained attention and impulse control in hyperactive and normal children. Can. J. Behav. Sci. 4:259–282.

Douglas, V. I. 1974. Sustained attention and impulse control: Implications for the handicapped child. In J. A. Swets and L. L. Elliot (eds.), Psychology and the Handicapped Child. U.S. Office of Education, Washington, D.C.

Douglas, V. I. 1975. Are drugs enough?—To treat or to train the hyperactive child. Int. J. Ment. Health 4:199–212.

Douglas, V. I., Parry, P., Marton, P., and Garson, C. 1976. Assessment of a cognitive training program for hyperactive children. J. Abnorm. Child Psychol. 4:389–410.

Dubey, D. R. 1976. Organic factors in hyperkinesis: A critical evaluation. Am. J. Orthopsychiatry 47:353–366.

Dubey, D. R., Kaufman, K. F., and O'Leary S. G. 1977a. Behavioral and reflective parent training for hyperactive children: A comparison. Paper presented at the 85th Annual Convention of the American Psychological Association, August 26, San Francisco, California.

Dubey, D. R., Kaufman, K. F. and O'Leary, S. G. 1977b. Training parents of hyperactive children in child management: A comparative outcome study. Unpublished manuscript State University of New York at Stony Brook.

Eysenck, H., and Rachman, S. T. 1971. The application of learning theory to child psychiatry. In T. C. Howells (ed.), Modern Perspectives in Child Psychiatry, pp. 104–169. Brunner/Mazel, New York.

Fagot, B. I., and Patterson, G. R. 1969. An in vivo analysis of reinforcing contingencies for sex-role behaviors in the pre-school child. Dev. Psychol. 1:563–568.

Feighner, A. 1975. Videotape learning for parents as therapeutic agents with hyperactive children. In D. P. Cantwell (ed.), The Hyperactive Child: Diagnosis, Management, Current Research, pp. 145–157. Halsted Press, New York.

Feighner, A. C., and Feighner, J. P. 1974. Multimodality treatment of the hyperactive child. Am. J. Psychiatry. 131:459–463.

Finch, A. J., Wilkinson, M. D., Nelson, W. M., and Montgomery, L. E. 1975. Modification of an impulsive cognitive tempo in emotionally disturbed boys. J. Abnorm. Child Psychol. 3:49–52.

Firestone, P., and Douglas, V. I. 1975. The effects of reward and punishment on reaction times and autonomic activity in hyperactive and normal children. J. Abnorm. Child Psychol. 3:201–216.

Firestone, P., and Douglas, V. I. 1977. The effects of verbal and material rewards and punishers on the performance of impulsive and reflective children. Child Study J. 7:71–78.

Forehand, R., and Atkeson, B. M. 1977. Generality of treatment effects with parents as therapists: A review of assessment and implementation procedures. Behav. Ther. 8:575–593.

Forehand, R., and Wells, K. C. 1977. Teachers and parents: Where have all the "good" contingency managers gone? Behav. Ther. 8:1010.

Franks, C. M., and Wilson, G. T. 1974. Annual Review of Behavior Therapy: Theory and Practice, Vol. 2. Brunner/Mazel, New York.

Franks, C. M., and Wilson, G. T. 1975. Annual Review of Behavior Therapy: Theory and Practice, Vol. 3. Brunner/Mazel, New York.

Franks, C. M., and Wilson, G. T. 1976. Annual Review of Behavior Therapy: Theory and Practice, Vol. 4. Brunner/Mazel, New York.

Franks, C. M., and Wilson, G. T. 1977. Annual Review of Behavior Therapy: Theory and Practice, Vol. 5. Brunner/Mazel, New York.

Freibergs, V., and Douglas, V. I. 1969. Concept learning in hyperactive and normal children. J. Abnorm. Psychol. 74:388–395.

Furman, S., and Feighner, A. 1973. Video feedback in treating hyperkinetic children: A preliminary report. Am. J. Psychiatry 130:790–796.

Gittelman-Klein, R., and Klein, D. 1975. Are behavioral and psychometric changes related in methylphenidate-treated, hyperactive children? Int. J. Ment. Health 4:182–198.

Gittelman-Klein, R., Klein, D. F., Abikoff, H., Katz, S., Gloisten, A. C., and Kates, W. 1976. Relative efficacy of methylphenidate and behavior modification in hyperkinetic children: An interim report. J. Abnorm. Child Psychol. 4:361–379.

Goldfried, M. R., and Davison, G. C. 1976. Clinical Behavior Therapy. Holt, Rinehart & Winston, Inc., New York.

Goldfried, M. R. and Merbaum, M. 1974. Behavior Change Through Self-Control. Holt, Rinehart, & Winston, Inc., New York.

Goldiamond, I. A. 1974. Towards a constructional approach to social problems. Behaviorism 2:1–85.

Gordon, T. 1970. P. E. T.: Parent Effectiveness Training. Wyden, New York.

Graziano, A. M. 1977. Parents as behavior therapists. In M. Hersen, R. M. Eisler, and P. M. Miller (eds.), Progress in Behavior Modification: Volume 4. Academic Press, New York.

Haight, M. J., Irvine, A. B., and Jampolsky, G. G. 1976. The response of hyperkinesis to EMG biofeedback. Paper presented at the meeting of the Biofeedback Research Society. Colorado Springs, Colorado.

Hall, R. V., Lund, D., and Jackson, D. 1968. Effects of teacher attention on study behavior. J. Appl. Behav. Anal. 1:1–12.

Hartmann, D. P., Roper, B. L., and Gelfand, D. M. 1977. An evaluation of alternative modes of child psychotherapy. In B. B. Lahey and A. E. Kazdin (eds.), Advances in Clinical Child Psychology, Vol. 1, pp. 1–46. Plenum Publishing Corp., New York.

Hastings, J. E., and Barkley, R. A. 1978. A review of psychophysiological research with hyperactive children. J. Abnorm. Child Psychol. 6:413–447.

Hersen, M., and Barlow, D. H. 1976. Single Case Experimental Designs: Strategies for Studying Behavior Change. Pergamon Press, Inc., New York.

Higa, W. R. 1973. Self-instructional versus direct training in modifying children's impulsive behavior. Unpublished doctoral dissertation, University of Hawaii.

Holland, C. J. 1970. An interview guide for behavioral counseling with parents. Behav. Ther. 1:70–79.

Huessy, H. R., Metoyer, M., and Townsend, M. 1974. 8–10 year follow-up of 84 children treated for behavioral disorder in rural Vermont. Acta Paedopsychiatr. 40:230–235.

Humphries, T., Kinsbourne, M., and Swanson, J. 1978. Stimulant effects on cooperation and social interaction between hyperactive children and their mothers. J. Child Psychol. Psychiatry 19:13–22.

Jacob, R. G., O'Leary, K. D., and Rosenblad, C. 1978. Formal and informal classroom settings: Effects on hyperactivity. J. Abnorm. Child Psychol. 6:47–59.

Johnson, C., and Katz, R. C. 1973. Using parents as change agents for their children: A review. J. Child Psychol. Psychiatry 14:181–200.

Johnson, S. M., Bolstad, O. D., and Lobitz, G. K. 1976. Generalization and contrast phenomena in behavior modification with children. In E. J. Mash, L. A. Hamerlynck, and L. C. Handy (eds.), Behavior Modification and Families, pp. 160–188. Brunner/Mazel, New York.

Kanfer, F. H., and Karoly, P. 1972. Self-control: A behavioristic excursion into the lion's den. Behav. Ther. 3:398–416.

Kazdin, A. E. 1973. The effect of vicarious reinforcement on attentive behavior in the classroom. J. Appl. Behav. Anal. 6:71–78.

Keeley, S. M., Shemberg, K. M., and Carbonell, J. 1976. Operant clinical intervention: Behavior management or legend? Where are the data? Behav. Ther. 7:292–305.

Kendall, P. C. 1977. On the efficacious use of verbal self-instructional procedures with children. Cognitive Ther. Res. 1:331–341.

Kendall, P. C., and Finch, A. J. 1976. A cognitive-behavioral treatment for impulse control: A case study. J. Consult. Clin. Psychol. 44:852–857.

Kendall, P. C., and Finch, A. J. 1978. A cognitive-behavioral treatment for impulsivity: A group comparison study. J. Consult. Clin. Psychol. 46:110–118.

Kiesler, D. J. 1971. Experimental designs in psychotherapy research. In A. E. Bergin and S. L. Garfield (eds.), Handbook of Psychotherapy and Behavior Change: An Empirical Analysis, pp. 36–74. John Wiley & Sons, Inc., New York.

Kistner, J. A. 1977. Attentional deficits of hyperkinetic children. Paper presented at the meeting of the Association for the Advancement of Behavior Therapy, December, Atlanta, Georgia.

Krasner, L. 1976. On the death of behavior modification: Some comments from a mourner. Am. Psychol. 31:387–388.

Lambert, N. M., Sandoval, J. H., and Sassone, D. M. 1977. Multiple prevalence estimates of hyperactivity in school children. Unpublished manuscript, University of California at Berkeley.

Langhorne, J. E., Loney, J., Paternite, C. E., and Bechtoldt, H. P. 1976. Childhood hyperkinesis: A return to the source. J. Abnorm. Psychol. 85:201–209.

London, P. 1972. The end of ideology in behavior modification. Am. Psychol. 27:913–920.

Loney, J., Comly, H., and Simon, B. 1975. Parental management, self-concept, and drug response in minimal brain dysfunction. J. Learn. Disabil. 8:187–190.

Loney, J., Langhorne, J. E., Paternite, C. E., Whaley-Klahn, M. A., Broeker, C. T., and Hacker, M. 1976. The Iowa HABIT: Hyperkinetic/aggressive boys in treatment. Paper presented at the meeting of the Society for Life History Research in Psychopathology, Fort Worth, Texas.

Lovaas, O. I., Koegel, R. L., Simmons, J. Q., and Long, J. S. 1973. Some generalization and follow-up measures on autistic children in behavior therapy. J. Appl. Behav. Anal. 6:131–165.

Lubar, J. F., and Shouse, M. N. 1976. EEG and behavioral changes in a hyperkinetic child concurrent with training of the sensorimotor rhythm (SMR); A preliminary report. Biofeedback and Self-Regulation 1:293–301.

Lubar, J. F., and Shouse, M. N. 1977. Use of biofeedback in the treatment of seizure disorders and hyperactivity. In B. B. Lahey and A. E. Kazdin (eds.) Advances in Clinical Child Psychology, Vol. 1, pp. 203–265. Plenum Publishing Corp., New York.

Luria, A. R. 1961. The Role of Speech in the Regulation of Normal and Abnormal Behavior. Liveright, New York.

Mahoney, M. M. 1974. Cognition and Behavior Modification. Ballinger, Cambridge, Mass.

Mahoney, M. J., Kazdin, A. E., and Lesswing, N. J. 1974. Behavior modification: Delusion or deliverance? In C. M. Franks and G. T. Wilson (eds.), Annual Review of Behavior Therapy: Theory and Practice, Vol. 2, pp. 11–40. Bruner/Mazel, New York.

Marwit, S. J., and Stenner, A. J. 1972. Hyperkinesis: Delineation of two patterns. Except. Child. 38:401–406.

Mash, E. J. 1976. Behavior modification and methodology: A developmental perspective. J. Educat. Thought 10:5–21.

Mash, E. J., Hamerlynck, L. A., and Handy, L. C. 1976. Behavior Modification and Families. Brunner/Mazel, New York.

Mash, E. J., Handy, L. C., and Hamerlynck, L. A. 1976. Behavior Modification Approaches to Parenting. Brunner/Mazel, New York.

Mash, E. J., and McElwee, J. D. 1976. Manual for coding interactions. In E. J. Mash and L. G. Terdal (eds.), Behavior Therapy Assessment: Diagnosis, Design and Evaluation, pp. 309–333. Springer, New York.

Mash, E. J., and McElwee, J. D. 1978. Videotape behavioral parent training: A group comparison. Unpublished manuscript, University of Calgary.

Mash, E. J., and Mercer, B. J. 1979. A comparison of the behavior of deviant and nondeviant boys while playing alone and interacting with a sibling. J. Child Psychol. Psychiatry. In press.

Mash, E. J., and Sinclair, C. 1977. Cognitive versus social-behavioral training in the generalization of a self-instructional program for impulsive children. Unpublished manuscript, University of Calgary.

Mash, E. J., and Terdal, L. G. 1976. Behavior Therapy Assessment: Diagnosis, Design and Evaluation. Springer, New York.

Mash, E. J., and Terdal, L. G. 1977. After the dance is over: Some issues and suggestions for follow-up assessment in behavior therapy. Psychol. Rep. 41:1287–1308.

Mash, E. J., and Terdal, L. G. 1979. Issues in the assessment of behavioral persistence. In P. Karoly and J. Steffen (eds.), Sources of Long-Term Change in Psychotherapy. Gardner Press, New York. In press.

Mash, E. J., Terdal, L. G., and Anderson, K. A. 1973. The response-class matrix: A procedure for recording parent-child interactions. J. Consult. Clin. Psychol. 40:163–164.

Meichenbaum, D. 1974. Cognitive-Behavior Modification. General Learning Press, Morristown, N.J.

Meichenbaum, D. 1977. Cognitive-Behavior Modification. Plenum Publishing Corp., New York.

Meichenbaum, D., and Goodman, J. 1969a. Reflection-impulsivity and verbal control of motor behavior. Child Dev. 40:785–797.

Meichenbaum, D., and Goodman, J. 1969b. The developmental control of operant motor responding by verbal operants. J. Exp. Child Psychol. 7:553–565.

Meichenbaum, D., and Goodman, J. 1971. Training impulsive children to talk to themselves: A means of developing self-control. J. Abnorm. Psychol. 77:115–126.

Mendelson, W., Johnson, N., and Stewart, M. A. 1971. Hyperactive children as teenagers: A follow-up study. J. Nerv. Ment. Dis. 153:273–279.

Miller, W. H. 1975. Systematic Parent Training. Research Press, Champaign, Ill.

Mischel, W. 1973. Toward a cognitive social learning reconceptualization of personality. Psychol. Rev. 80:252–283.

Nall, A. 1973. Alpha training and the hyperkinetic child: Is it effective? Academ. Ther. 9:5–19.

Ney, P. G. 1974. Four types of hyperkinesis. Can. Psychiatr. Assoc. J. 19:543–550.

Nixon, S. B. 1969. Increasing task-oriented behavior. In J. D. Krumboltz and C. E. Thoresen (eds.), Behavioral Counseling: Cases and Techniques, pp. 207–210. Holt, Rinehart & Winston, Inc., New York.

O'Dell, S. 1974. Training parents in behavior modification: A review. Psychol. Bull. 81:418–433.

O'Leary, K. D., and O'Leary, S. G. 1972. Classroom Management: The Successful Use of Behavior Modificaton. Pergamon Press, Inc., New York.

O'Leary, K. D., Pelham, W. E., Rosenbaum, A., and Price, G. H. 1976. Behavioral treatment of hyperkinetic children: An experimental evaluation of its usefulness. Clin. Pediatr. 15:510–515.

O'Leary, S. G. 1977. Behavioral treatment of hyperactive children. Paper presented at the annual meeting of the Association for the Advancement of Behavior Therapy, December, Atlanta, Georgia.

O'Leary, S. G., and Pelham, W. E. 1978. Behavior therapy and withdrawal of stimulant medication in hyperactive children. Pediatrics. 61:211–217.

Palkes, H., Stewart, M., and Freedman, J. 1972. Improvement in maze performance of hyperactive boys as a function of verbal-training procedures. J. Special Educ. 5:337–342.

Palkes, H., Stewart, M., and Kahana, B. 1968. Porteus Maze performance of hyperactive boys after training in self-directed commands. Child Dev. 39:817–826.

Parry, P., and Douglas, V. I. 1973. The effect of reward on the performance of hyperactive children. Diss. Abstr. Int. 34:6220B.

Paternite, M. A., Loney, J., and Langhorne, J. E. 1976. Relationships between symptomatology and SES-related factors in hyperkinetic/MBD boys. Am. J. Orthopsychiatry 46:291–301.

Patterson, G. R. 1965. An application of conditioning techniques to the control of a hyperactive child. In L. P. Ullman and L. Krasner (eds.), Case Studies in Behavior Modification, pp. 370–375. Holt, Rinehart and Winston, Inc., New York.

Patterson, G. R. 1976. The aggressive child: Victim and architect of a coercive system. In E. J. Mash, L. A. Hamerlynck, and L. C. Handy (eds.), Behavior Modification and Families, pp. 267–316. Brunner/Mazel, New York.

Patterson, G. R., Jones, R., Whittier, J., and Wright, M. A. 1965. A behavior modification technique for the hyperactive child. Behav. Res. Ther. 2:217–226.

Patterson, G. R., Ray, R. S., Shaw, D. A., and Cobb, J. A. 1969. Manual for coding family interactions, sixth revision. Available from ASIS National Auxiliary Publications Service Inc., 909 Third Avenue, New York, N.Y., 10022. Document No. 01234.

Patterson, G. R., Reid, J. B., Jones, R. R., and Conger, R. E. 1975. A Social Learning Approach to Family Intervention. Castalia, Eugene, Ore.

Pelham, W. E. 1976. Behavioral treatment of hyperkinesis. Am. J. Dis. Child. 130:565.

Pelham, W. E. 1977. Withdrawal of a stimulant drug and concurrent behavioral intervention in the treatment of a hyperactive child. Behav. Ther. 8:473–479.

Pelham, W. E. 1978. Hyperactive children. Psychiatr. Clin. North Am. 1:227–245.

Pihl, R. 1967. Conditioning procedures with hyperactive children. Neurology 17:421–423.

Prout, H. T. 1977. Behavioral intervention with hyperactive children. A review. J. Learn. Disabil. 10:141–146.

Putre, W., Loffio, K., Chorost, S., Marx, V., and Gilbert, C. 1977. An effectiveness study of a relaxation training tape with hyperactive children. Behav. Ther. 8:355–359.

Rapoport, J. L., and Benoit, M. 1975. The relation of direct home observations to the clinic evaluation of hyperactive school-age boys. J. Child Psychol. Psychiatry 16:141–147.

Reisinger, J. J., Ora, J. P., and Frangia, G. W. 1976. Parents as change agents for their children: A review. J. Community Psychol. 4:103–123.

Rie, E. D., and Rie, H. 1977. Recall, retention and Ritalin. J. Consult. Clin. Psychol. 45:967–972.

Rie, H. E., Rie, E. D., Stewart, S., and Ambuel, J. P. 1976a. Effects of methylphenidate on underachieving children. J. Consult. Clin. Psychol. 44:250–260.

Rie, H. E., Rie, E. D., Stewart, S., and Ambuel, J. P. 1976b. Effects of Ritalin on underachieving children: A replication. Am. J. Orthopsychiatry 46:313–322.

Risley, T. R. 1968. Behavior modification: An experimental therapeutic endeavor. In L. A. Hamerlynck, P. O. Davidson, and L. E. Acker (eds.), Behavior Modification and Ideal Mental Health Services, pp. 103–127. University of Calgary, Calgary, Alberta, Canada.

Risley, T. R. 1977. Winning. Presidential address to the Association for the Advancement of Behavior Therapy, December, Atlanta, Georgia.

Rosenbaum, A., O'Leary, K. D., and Jacob, R. G. 1975. Behavioral intervention with hyperactive children: Group consequences as a supplement to individual contingencies. Behav. Ther. 6:315–323.

Ross, A. 1976. Psychological Aspects of Learning Disabilities and Reading Disorders. McGraw-Hill Book Company, New York.

Ross, D. M., and Ross, S. A. 1976. Hyperactivity: Research, Theory and Action. John Wiley & Sons, New York.

Routh, D. K., Schroeder, C. S., and O'Tuama, L. A. 1974. Development of activity level in children. Dev. Psychol. 10:163–168.

Rutter, M. 1977. Brain damage syndromes in childhood: Concepts and findings. J. Child Psychol. Psychiatry 18:1–21.

Ryback, D., and Staats, A. W. 1970. Parents as behavior therapy technicians in treating reading deficits (dyslexia). J. Behav. Ther. Exp. Psychiatry 1:109–119.

Sachs, D. A. 1973. The efficacy of time-out procedures in a variety of behavior problems. J. Behav. Ther. Exp. Psychiatry 4:237–242.

Safer, D., and Allen, R. 1976. Hyperactive Children: Diagnosis and Management. University Park Press, Baltimore.

Schleifer, M., Weiss, G., Cohen, N., Elman, M., Cvejic, H., and Kruger, E. 1975. Hyperactivity in preschoolers and the effect of methylphenidate. Am. J. Orthopsychiatry 45:38–50.

Shrager, J., and Lindy, J. 1970. Hyperkinetic children: Early indicators of potential school failure. Community Ment. Health J. 6:447–454.

Seitz, S., and Terdal, L. 1972. A modeling approach to changing parent-child interactions. Ment. Retard. 4:39–43.

Shafto, F., and Sulzbacher, S. 1977. Comparing treatment tactics with a hyperactive preschool child: Stimulant medication and programmed teacher intervention. J. Appl. Behav. Anal. 10:13–20.

Sidman, M. 1960. Tactics of Scientific Research: Evaluating Experimental Data in Psychology. Basic Books, Inc., New York.

Simmons, J. Q. 1975. Behavioral management of the hyperactive child. In D. P. Cantwell (ed.), The Hyperactive Child: Diagnosis, Management, Current Research, pp. 129–143. Halsted Press, New York.

Simpson, D. D., and Nelson, A. E. 1972. Breathing Control and Attention Training: A Preliminary Study of a Psychophysiological Approach to Self-Control of Hyperactive Behavior in Children. Texas Christian University, Institute of Behavior Research, Fort Worth, Texas.

Skindrud, K. D. 1972. Generalization of treatment effects from home to school settings. Unpublished manuscript, Oregon Research Institute.

Sprague, R. L., Cohen, M., and Werry, J. S. 1974. Normative data on the Conners Teacher Rating Scale and Abbreviated Scale. Children's Research Center, Technical Report, November. University of Illinois, Urbana-Champaign.

Sprague, R. L., and Sleator, E. K. 1977. Methylphenidate in hyperkinetic children: Differences in dose effects on learning and social behavior. Science 198:1274–1276.

Sprague, R. L., and Werry, J. S. 1971. Methodology of psychopharmacological studies with the retarded. In N. R. Ellis (ed.), International Review of Research in Mental Retardation, pp. 147–219. Academic Press, New York.

Sroufe, L. A. 1975. Drug treatment of children with behavior problems. In F. D. Horowitz (ed.), Review of Child Development Research, Vol. 4, pp. 347–407. University of Chicago Press, Chicago, Ill.

Strong, C., Sulzbacher, S. I., and Kirkpatrick, M. A. 1974. Use of medication versus reinforcement to modify a classroom behavior disorder. J. Learn. Disabil. 7:214–218.

Sulzbacher, S. I. 1972. Behavior analysis of drug effects in the classroom. In G. Samb (ed.), Behavior Analysis and Education—1972, pp. 37–52. University of Kansas, Lawrence. (1973)

Sulzbacher, S. I. 1973. Psychotropic medication with children: An evaluation of procedural biases in results of reported studies. Pediatrics 51:513–517.

Sulzbacher, S. I. 1975. The learning disabled or hyperactive child: Diagnosis and treatment. J.A.M.A. 234:938–941.

Swanson, J. M., and Kinsbourne, M. 1976. Stimulant-related state-dependent learning in hyperactive children. Science 192:1354–1357.

Tharp, R. G., and Wetzel, R. J. 1969. Behavior Modification in the Natural Environment. Academic Press, New York.

Thomas, G. M. 1974. Using videotaped modeling to increase attending behavior. Elementary School Guidance and Counseling 9:35–50.

Thoreson, C. E., and Mahoney, M. J. 1974. Behavioral Self-Control. Holt, Rinehart & Winston, Inc., New York.

Twardosz, S., and Sajwaj, T. 1972. Multiple effects of a procedure to increase sitting in a hyperactive, retarded boy. J. Appl. Behav. Anal. 5:73–78.

Ullman, L. P., and Krasner, L. (eds.) 1965. Case Studies in Behavior Modification. Holt, Rinehart & Winston, Inc., New York.

Varni, J. W., and Henker, B. 1978. A self-regulation approach to the treatment of the hyperactive child. Behav. Ther. In press.

Wahler, R. G. 1975. Some structural aspects of deviant child behavior. J. Appl. Behav. Anal. 8:27–42.

Wahler, R. G., Berland, R. M., Coe, T. D., and Leske, G. 1977. Social systems analysis: Implementing an alternative behavioral model. In A. Rogers-Warren and S. F. Warren (eds.), Ecological Perspectives in Behavior Analysis, pp. 211–228. University Park Press, Baltimore.

Wahler, R. G., House, A. E., and Stambaugh, E. E. 1976. Ecological Assessment of Child Problem Behavior: A Clinical Package for Home, School and Institutional Settings. Pergamon Press, Inc., New York.

Waldrop, M. F., Bell, R. Q., McLaughlin, B., and Halverson, C. F. 1978. Newborn minor physical anomalies predict short attention span, peer aggression, and impulsivity at age 3. Science 199:563–565.

Weiss, G., Minde, K., Werry, J. S., Douglas, V. I., and Nemeth, E. 1971. Studies on the hyperactive child: VIII. Five-year follow-up. Arch. Gen. Psychiatry 24:409–414.

Wender, P. H. 1971. Minimal Brain Dysfunction in Children. Wiley-Interscience, New York.

Werry, J. S. 1968. Developmental hyperactivity. Pediatr. Clin. North Am. 15:581–599.

Werry, J. S., and Sprague, R. L. 1970. Hyperactivity. In C. G. Costello (ed.), Symptoms of Psychopathology: A Handbook, pp. 397–417. John Wiley & Sons, Inc., New York.

Whalen, C. K., and Henker, B. 1976. Psychostimulants and children: A review and analysis. Psychol. Bull. 83:1113–1130.

Williams, B., and Vincent, J. 1977. HABOS: Code system for hyperactivity. Unpublished manuscript, Baylor School of Medicine and University of Houston.

Williams, B. J., Vincent, J., and Elrod, J. T. 1977. Preliminary draft of the behavioral components of hyperactivity. Paper presented at the annual meeting of the American Psychological Association, August, San Francisco, California.

Willis, T. J., and Lovaas, I. 1977. A behavioral approach to treating hyperactive children: The parent's role. In J. G. Millichap (ed.), Learning Disabilities and Related Disorders: Facts and Current Issues. Year Book Medical Publishers, Chicago, Ill.

Wolpe, J. 1969. The Practice of Behavior Therapy. Pergamon, Oxford.

Wolraich, M. L. 1977. Stimulant drug therapy in hyperactive children: Research and clinical implications. Pediatrics 60:512–518.

Wolraich, M., Drummond, T., Salomon, M. K., O'Brien, M. L., and Sivage, C. 1978. Effects of methylphenidate alone and in combination with behavior modification procedures on the behavior and academic performance of hyperactive children. J. Abnorm. Child Psychol. 6:149–161.

Worland, J. 1976. Effects of positive and negative feedback on behavior control in hyperactive and normal boys. J. Abnorm. Child Psychol. 4:315–326.

Wulbert, M., and Dries, R. 1977. The relative efficacy of methylphenidate (Ritalin) and behavior modification techniques in the treatment of a hyperactive child. J. Appl. Behav. Anal. 10:21–31.

Zivin, G. 1974. How to make a boring thing more boring. Child Dev. 45:232–236.

Assessment
of Intervention

Robert L. Sprague

THE IMPORTANCE OF ASSESSMENT METHODOLOGY

There is a vast literature on hyperactivity, and it is growing at a cancerous rate (Wender, 1971, 1973; Stewart and Olds, 1973; Renshaw, 1974; Cantwell, 1975; Schrag and Divoky, 1975; Winchell, 1975; Ross and Ross, 1976; Safer and Allen, 1976; Bosco and Robin, 1977; Kirson, Lipman, and Reatig, 1978). Although one might normally expect that such a large literature would reflect a major body of empirical knowledge, this is not the case because so many of the studies are methodologically weak, unsophisticated, or blatantly biased (Freeman, 1970, 1976; Sprague and Werry, 1971, 1974). Such a mass of confusing, contradictory, and misleading literature confounds not only the general public but also researchers in the area.

I can think of no better example of the confusion generated by this literature than citing my yearly experience teaching a graduate seminar in special education on the topic of Drugs in Special Education (Sprague and Gadow, 1977). The course is taken by graduate students who represent a number of different backgrounds: special education teachers who are coming back to the university for advanced training, classroom teachers who are taking advanced training to prepare themselves for special education, graduate students from allied departments, e.g., psychology, who are interested in the general issue of psychopharmacology of children, and graduate students in special education who have not taught in the schools. Over 97% of special education teachers who have experience teaching children in special education classes have encountered a child in their class who was receiving psychoactive or anticonvulsant drugs (Gadow, 1978). In fact, 86% have experience with a

Preparation of this paper was supported in part by PHS Grant No. MH18909 from the National Institute of Mental Health.

child receiving psychoactive medication for hyperactivity. On the basis of their first-hand experience, they have some limited information about how the drugs may influence the behavior of children receiving the medication. Nevertheless, there are vast gaps in their knowledge because it is only as good, obviously, as the comprehensiveness of their personal experience. There is a tremendous gap in terms of knowledge about psychoactive drugs between what special education teachers experience in the classroom and what they are prepared for by their formal training (Sprague and Gadow, 1977). We routinely encounter teachers who confuse the side effects of psychopharmacologic agents with the child's behavior problem. For example, the well-known sedating effects of the commonly used neuroleptic (tranquilizing) drugs for behavior disorders are sometimes interpreted as lack of motivation and disinterest on the part of the child. Furthermore, teachers are often unduly influenced by the less well documented and studied interventions of fads such as fluorescent lights, sugar intake, etc.

In a highly critical paper, Freeman (1976) wrote on the topic of "Minimal Brain Dysfunction, Hyperactivity, and Learning Disorders: Epidemic or Episode?" One of the main themes of the paper is that because of the fuzziness of the diagnosis of minimal brain dysfunction and hyperactivity, writers have postulated causes at an epidemic rate. For example, he lists the following as possible causes: anoxia, maturational lag, allergy, maternal smoking, genetics, temperament, visual problems, fluorescent lights, subclinical lead intoxication, starvation, and a very broad, general class of causes known as psychosocial factors. Accompanying the epidemic of causes, he also listed an epidemic of cures, treatments, or interventions. It is quite clear from Freeman's paper that such a situation can exist because interventions have not been critically and scientifically evaluated with methodologically sound experiments; consequently misinterpretation, overgeneralizations, and excess enthusiasm have pushed out cautious, critical evaluations just as bad money drives out good money in an economic crisis.

As examples of the more faddish treatments that have been suggested for hyperactivity, two treatments will be discussed. In a brief news article, Arehart-Treichel (1974) uncritically reported on the filming of one child in one Florida classroom by the Environmental Health and Light Research Institute in Florida. It was suggested in the news release that x-rays emanating from the cathode ends of fluorescent tubes might cause hyperactivity. Approximately 2 years later, a brief report of the case study was made by Ott (1976). If one assumes even minimal methodological standards (Sprague and Werry, 1971), it is clear that this case study is woefully inadequate. Nevertheless, Ott drew firm conclusions from the case study, as evidenced by this quote, "Under improved lighting conditions, using full-spectrum fluorescent tubes with lead foil shields over the cathode ends of the fluorescent to stop soft x-rays, children's behavior in the classroom showed *dramatic improvement*" (italics added). Now what is the "dramatic improvement" based on?

First, special cameras "out of view of the children" were mounted near the ceiling in the classroom to film the children. Nothing is said about obtaining the informed consent of the school, the teacher, or the parents of the children to film in the classroom, although the current climate of concern about human subjects is obvious to most researchers (Katz, 1972; Hershey and Miller, 1976; Sprague, 1978). Second, the experimental conditions are vaguely described—"lead foil shields were wrapped around the cathode ends of the tubes to stop suspected soft x-rays." Third, the casual analysis was based on 13 photographs, published in the article, that primarily focused on one boy usually seated at a table in the classroom. There is no description of when the photographs were taken or of the conditions in the classroom during the filming. Fourth, there were no control conditions, i.e., randomized use of ordinary fluorescent tubes and shielded tubes during some extended period of time. Fifth, there was no random assignment of the subjects to conditions since there was only one subject. Sixth, there is not even a hint in the article as to whether double-blind conditions were used—i.e., keeping the nature of the experiment confidential from people interpreting the situation, such as the teacher and observers, if any. In fact, a film on the topic viewed by the author seems to indicate that the shielded fluorescent tubes were installed at the same time that the target boy was reassigned a seat adjacent to the teacher's desk. Nevertheless, the interpretation was made that the shielded tubes were more influential on changing the child's behavior than the close proximity to the teacher's desk. Finally, there was no statistical analysis, nor was there any comparison with other possible interventions for hyperactivity to yield empirical data about the relative effect of the shielded fluorescent tubes.

In stark contrast to the case study cited above, a methodologically sound experiment has been conducted by O'Leary, Rosenbaum, and Hughes (1978). In this study, the conditions were highly specified, including the exact kind and type of fluorescent light and the type of shields. Listing our minimum methodological criteria (Sprague and Werry, 1971), the following standards were met:

1. The children served as their own controls.
2. An alternating schedule of lighting conditions was established weekly during an 8-week period.

3. Great care was taken to ensure that people important to the outcome of the study, such as teacher and observers, were blind as to the lighting conditions.

4. Quite specific standardized procedures for both the shielded and the unshielded lights were used throughout the experiment.

5. A standardized evaluation consisting of a specified observation schedule with data about its reliability was used.

6. Appropriate analyses of variance were calculated on the data; the results indicated that there was no effect resulting from the change in fluorescent lights.

It has been suggested that simply by introducing background music in the classroom, hyperactivity may be controlled (Scott, 1970; Pepper, 1974). Rather than again enumerating the minimum methodologic criteria point by point, only weaknesses of the study (Scott, 1970) will be discussed. Only four subjects were used. They were diagnosed (no criteria given) as "hyperactive" and as showing evidence of "minimal brain injury." Nothing was said about double-blind conditions or how the teachers were informed as to the nature of the study. The standarized evaluations left something to be desired. The measurement of performance change was simply described as a deck of cards containing arithmetic problems appropriate to the level of achievement. Finally a statistical analysis was done (Friedman two-way analysis of variance) that was found to show significant differences. It was stated that the results ". . . confirm the observation that productivity of hyperactive children in an academic setting may be enhanced by the introduction of background music." However, the data for the four experimental conditions showed that the average number of correct arithmetic problems varied with the presence of background music as much as it did without background music (29.8 with music in a booth versus 46.3 with music in the classroom in comparison with 38.7 without music in a booth versus 26.7 without music in the classroom).

For whatever reasons, the article on music has not led to a national campaign to install Muzak in our schools, whereas some of the other fads have resulted in such undertakings. An effort has been underway to convince the United States Congress that legislation should be passed with the necessary millions in appropriations to convert all the old fluorescent light fixtures in schools to the shielded type. Such efforts at political pressure based on simplistic, methodologically unsound case studies are, at the very best, premature and seriously damaging to the general public's faith in the credibility of research-derived information.

ASSESSMENT MODELS

Several schema or models have been developed for assessing the effectiveness of intervention procedures in children's behavioral disorders. The most highly refined and sophisticated set of measures developed are derived from the area of pediatric psychopharmacology, possibly because there are more controversies regarding the efficacy of drug intervention, thus requiring more time and effort to be devoted to developing evaluation procedures.

About 7 years ago, we reviewed a large body of literature regarding the psychopharmacology of mentally retarded people and listed six minimum criteria for evaluating intervention studies (Sprague and Werry, 1971). The criteria are:

1. Placebo control
2. Random assignment of subjects
3. Double-blind conditions
4. Standardized dosages
5. Standardized evaluations
6. Appropriate statistical analyses

Placebo control means that there must be a control condition differing from the treatment condition only in that the intervention is not administered during the control. In other words, the control is a baseline condition against which behavior can be assessed with respect to the changes observed under the intervention condition. Since most of the intervention procedures for hyperactivity are new or relatively untried, it seems absolutely essential that a control or a placebo condition be used in studies attempting to assess the effectiveness of interventions.

From the standpoint of both statistical analysis and good experimental design, it is necessary to randomly assign subjects to conditions. In the typical between-groups experimental design, subjects are randomly assigned to one of the intervention groups. In a cross-over or within-subjects design, the subjects should be randomly or systematically (e.g., Latin square design) assigned to the sequence of conditions that will be administered. Other approaches to this problem of sequence or order effects raise questions that are difficult or impossible to answer after the experiment has been conducted. One of the experiments cited above used an alternating schedule of assigning the sequence of conditions. Such a procedure is less desirable than randomly determining the order.

Double-blind conditions exist when neither the subject involved nor the person evaluating the intervention is aware of which is the control condition and which is the active intervention. This procedure prevents the investigators' expectations and hopes from influencing their assessment of the behavioral changes, if any.

Standardized dosages in the pediatric psychopharmacological study simply means that the powerful variable of dosage must be standardized or controlled in some fashion rather than allowed to vary over individual subjects. When one allows such important variables to vary over subjects, there is complete confounding of this variable with the variations of individual subjects in such a fashion that it is impossible to disentangle the two. Such confoundings have produced many erroneous statistical evaluations and interpretations of data. In the more general case of assessment of intervention, this criterion means that the intervention must be applied in some known quantitative amount. If the intervention consists of psychoeducational training, then the training should be applied, for example, for a fixed period of time. If the intervention involves dietary manipulation, then the amount and quality of the dietary intervention should be specified in keeping with sound research practices of nutrition science.

Standardized evaluations mean that there must be some method of measurement that has been used before and/or for which empirical information on basic reliability and validity is available. In all too many cases in the hyperactivity area an intervention procedure has been evaluated by a measuring instrument developed explicitly for that experiment, without any information about its reliability, validity, or sensitivity.

Appropriate statistical analyses means simply what it says. Many textbooks have been written on this topic, and statistics will not be discussed here other than to say that the mere application of a statistical test does not necessarily sanctify the results and make them credible.

Since the publication of this 1971 article, we have added a seventh criterion (Sprague and Baxley, 1978). This seventh criterion involves comparing the intervention with some well-known treatment technique to obtain comparative efficacy information. This may not seem like an important point, but when the intervention concerns a dysfunction that may involve thousands or tens of thousands of children, then one must have empirical information about relative comparative efficacy. In the absence of such comparative information, erroneous judgments can be made about the cost/benefit ratios that might be obtained with some new or highly advertised intervention. Again, a very good example of this problem can be obtained from the pediatric psychopharmacology area. As Stewart (1975) has cogently argued, the treatment of enuresis in children is plagued with the problem of lack of comparative data. There are basically two intervention procedures for enuretic children: the conditioning procedure using the buzzer blanket, and the antidepressant drug imipramine. The effectiveness of the two treatment conditions are not equal. Stewart suggests that the behavioral therapy approach is probably 90% effective after one year has elapsed, whereas imipramine is probably 10% to 20% effective after 1 year. With such divergent outcome differences, one might think that the overwhelming choice of the intervention procedure would be the behavioral therapy approach. Not so! The most commonly used treatment procedure for enuretic children in the United States is prescription of imipramine. One might wonder why a less effective procedure is used, but one must consider the emphasis on biomedical procedures, e.g., drugs, by doctors in treating what is considered a disease (Engel, 1977; Muller, 1972). Besides the differences in efficacy, there are some very decided risks associated with the widespread use of imipramine, for example, a large increase in accidental poisoning of children (Parkin and Fraser, 1972). Thus, it should be quite apparent that the comparative intervention criterion can be, and often is, clinically very important.

There are a few sources for assessment models appropriate for the study of intervention in the hyperkinetic child syndrome. In 1973, the National Institute of Mental Health of the United States published a bulletin on the evaluation of pharmacotherapy with children (Sprague, 1973). Again, although this is devoted to psychopharmacology, much of the material is pertinent to the evaluation of intervention for hyperactivity. For example, the bulletin contains papers on these topics: a listing of rating scales and questionnaires that can be used to evaluate behavioral change in children, recommended performance measures, diagnosis for children, neurological examination, medical and social history, medical laboratory techniques, and rating of side effects.

The most thorough discussion in a single source of measures appropriate to evaluate intervention in hyperactivity can be found in a recently published book by Werry (1978b). In a chapter exclusively devoted to the problem of measures of the behavioral effects (1978a), Werry discusses the background of measurement, including such topics as reliability, validity, sensitivity, relevance, and other qualities of a test. In addition, he thoroughly reviews the sources of data: social contacts, observers, mechanical devices, self-report, etc. For anyone planning an assessment of interventions in hyperactive children, this chapter is highly recommended. In another important chapter in the same book that covers a topic often overlooked when evaluating interventions in hyperactivity, Aman (1978) discusses measures and designs to assess the effects of medication on learning performance in children. Since it is quite apparent that the task of the normal child is to go to school and learn, it seems that techniques and strategies to assess learning performance in children undergoing intervention techniques cannot be overemphasized.

In the above discussion of the effects of fluorescent lights on hyperactivity, it was mentioned that the consent of the subjects and the concern for the welfare of the children involved cannot be ignored, particularly in this day and age of concern about human rights. This is certainly true for interventions involving psychopharmacological techniques and for other interventions, as I have outlined in some detail (Sprague, 1978). Although in the past the experimenter had almost a free hand to determine the design, measuring techniques, and other aspects of the study, this is no longer true. In some cases the courts have determined that experimentation will not be permitted, and in other cases legislative bodies have sought to highly restrict certain kinds of experimentation (Brown and Bing, 1976).

ASSESSMENT OF BEHAVIORAL INTERVENTIONS

It might be assumed from the above discussion that many of the methodological assessment problems in this area are uniquely associated with psychopharmacological investigations, because the methodology of these studies has been referred to repeatedly. In order to dispel this impression, a discussion of methodological problems of assessing behavioral interventions in children's behavior disorders is in order. A good general source of information on behavioral assessment is Ciminero, Calhoun, and Adams (1977).

In an excellent paper that discussed most of the major methodologic pitfalls of behavior therapy evaluations, Kent and O'Leary (1976) outlined in some detail the methodological weaknesses of studies of behavioral therapy with problem children. They pointed out that there were several faults in previous studies:

1. ". . . the most serious limitation[s] was the absence of a matched control group or subjects randomly assigned to conditions. . ." in most of the studies.
2. ". . . the absence of reliable and objective measures of change obtained from persons other than the therapist or client."
3. ". . . absence of evidence indicating maintenance of behavioral improvements after termination of therapist contact."

4. Importance of multiple measures of academic as well as behavioral change.
5. A follow-up period of enough length to meaningfully assess the long-term efficacy.
6. A homogeneous population with regard to the diagnostic classification.

When these methodological points were met in a well-designed study conducted by Kent and O'Leary, the results were somewhat different than might be expected from the more enthusiastic supporters of behavioral therapy. In a composite measure of the disruptive behavior representing nine categories (interference with others, extended vocalization, noncompliance, physical aggression, verbal aggression, self-stimulation, daydreaming, solicitation of teacher attention, and off task), they found that, although there were significant differences at the termination of behavioral therapy between the treated and control children in favor, of course, of the treated children, these differences entirely disappeared after the passage of 9 months—". . . follow-up comparisons of treated and control children 9 months later provided a stark contrast with immediate effects of therapy." None of the nine categories or the composite were significantly different. In discussing the results, the authors warned that one must not make assumptions about long-term effects on the basis of short-term behavioral changes.

Often in evaluating the effects of an intervention technique, particularly in hyperactivity, the suppression of the symptoms of hyperactivity is unduly emphasized almost to the exclusion of other pertinent aspects, such as the ability of the child to learn (Sprague and Sleator, 1977). Perhaps part of this emphasis on symptom suppression as a single criterion of the effectiveness of intervention may be traced back to the inherent problems associated with the biomedical model (Engel, 1977). If one turns to other areas where controversies have existed about intervention, it is clear that such a simplistic criterion of improvement will no longer be satisfactory. In assessing the intervention efficacy of treatments with adult psychiatric patients, it has much too long been the case that the simplistic notion of suppression of the symptoms for the short and long term was the main consideration. In a thorough review of the literature of psychopharmacological treatment of schizophrenia from the standpoint of effects on prosocial behavior of adult psychiatric patients, Marholin and Phillips (1976) forcefully indicated that drug treatment effectively reduces or suppresses symptoms but seldom, if ever, enhances social behavior.

In other areas, such as the treatment of mentally retarded children, the emphasis on symptom suppression has led to a crisis that has resulted in extensive litigation in the court, legislation about the rights of the mentally retarded to treatment, and extensive regulation (Sprague, 1977; Sprague and Baxley, 1978). In fact, a new concept is rapidly gaining ascendency in the mental retardation area that replaces the simplistic notion of symptoms suppression. The concept of normalization, or enhancing the likelihood that the handicapped individual will be able to develop in a number of different behavioral areas to something near the maximum of his potential, has been expressed as a legal concept (Mason and Menolascino, 1976). This concept has been further strengthened by a court decision late in 1977 that expressed, in essence, the right of the mentally retarded individual to normalization or the right to habilitation (*Halderman* v. *Pennhurst*, 1977).

FUTURE ASSESSMENT PROCEDURES

The above discussion may be a rather dismal picture of the current status of assessment of interventions for hyperactivity, but there is every reason to believe that the future looks much better than the past. Besides considerable interest in the methodology of assessment of intervention and the publication of assessment models, there are some new techniques and procedures coming into the research marketplace that hold hope for the future.

There has always been the continuing problem of what to do clinically with the individual person who seems to be responding or reacting in a different manner than what the literature indicates should happen to groups of people in general. Most of the above discussion dealt with mean data for groups, but, of course, group data do not always accurately reflect the behavior of every member of the group, and certainly do not predict accurately the responses of individuals. In recent years, there has been a developing interest in procedures to assess the effects of experimental manipulations—interventions, if you will—on the single subject. A recent book (Hersen and Barlow, 1976) was devoted to this topic. I urge the use of such individual assessment procedures clinically after empirical group data have been developed. With the extensive interest in the field of hyperactivity, it seems that empirical data are being developed on groups; the next stage, the systematic study of individual cases, is important to consider and to begin.

Besides the renewed interest in individual cases, there is also unhappiness within the hyperactivity area about a single criterion for assessing improvement. Within the last year, some investigators (Vincent, Williams, and Elrod, 1977) have used the multitrait-multimethod to assess hyperactivity in classrooms, a technique that was first described by Campbell and Fiske in 1959. This approach looks particularly promising in studying the hyperactive child, because it should be obvious that hyperactivity is not a single behavioral expression but a complex constellation of a number of behavioral symptoms. It is urged that the most appropriate way to assess the effects of intervention in such a complicated syndrome is through use of the multitrait-multimethod technique.

SUMMARY

There has been much controversy in the area of hyperactivity, much premature touting of panaceas, perhaps an epidemic of causes (Freeman, 1976), and great confusion among the lay public as to what are appropriate interventions for these troubled children. Without apology, this paper has assumed a hard-headed experimental approach to the problem of assessing intervention. Some examples of farfetched causes and recommended interventions were given. A cogent example of cost/benefit judgments arising from the lack of comparative data on different intervention techniques was presented from the pediatric psychopharmacology area. Perhaps research and clinical workers will be encouraged to study the effects of combined behavioral, psychoeducational, and pharmacological interventions to help these children with their difficult problems.

REFERENCES

Aman, M. G. 1978. Drugs, learning and the psychotherapies. In J. S. Werry (ed.), Pediatric Psychopharmacology—The Use of Behavior Modifying Drugs in Children. Brunner/Mazel, New York.

Arehart-Treichel, J. 1974. School lights and problem pupils. Sci. News 105:258–259.

Bosco, J. J., and Robin, S. S. (eds.) 1977. The Hyperactive Child and Stimulant Drugs. University of Chicago Press, Chicago.

Brown, J. L., and Bing, S. R. 1976. Drugging children: Child abuse by professionals. In G. P. Koocher (ed.), Children's Rights and the Mental Health Professionals. John Wiley & Sons, Inc., New York.

Campbell, D. T., and Fiske, D. W. 1959. Convergent and discriminant validation by the multitrait–multi-method matrix. Psychol. Bull. 56:81–105.

Cantwell, D. P. 1975. The Hyperactive Child. Spectrum Publications, New York.

Ciminero, A. R., Calhoun, K. S., and Adams, H. E. 1977. Handbook of Behavioral Assessment. John Wiley & Sons, Inc., New York.

Engel, G. L. 1977. The need for a new medical model: A challenge for biomedicine. Science 196:129–136.

Freeman, R. D. 1970. Review of medicine in special education: Another look at drugs and behavior. J. Special Educ. 4:377–384.

Freeman, R. D. 1976. Minimal brain dysfunction, hyperactivity, and learning disorders: Epidemic or episode? School Rev. 85:5–30.

Gadow, K. D. 1978. Survey of medication usage with children in trainable mentally handicapped programs and teacher role in drug treatment. Doctoral dissertation, University of Illinois.

Halderman v. Pennhurst, No. 74-1345 (E.D. Pa. Dec. 23, 1977).

Hersen, M., and Barlow, D. H. 1976. Single-Case Experimental Designs: Strategies for Studying Behavior Change. Pergamon Press, Inc., New York.

Hershey, N., and Miller, R. D. 1976. Human Experimentation and the Law. Aspen Systems Corp., Germantown, Md.

Katz, J. 1972. Experimentation with Human Beings. Russell Sage Foundation, New York.

Kent, R. N., and O'Leary, K. D. 1976. A controlled evaluation of behavior modification with conduct problem children. J. Consult. Clin. Psychol. 44:586–596.

Kirson, T., Lipman, R., and Reatig, N. 1978. Bibliography on the Hyperkinetic Behavior Syndrome. (DHEW Publication No. (ADM) 77-449). U.S. Government Printing Office, Washington, D.C.

Marholin, D., II, and Phillips, D. 1976. Methodological issues in psychopharmacological research: Chlorpromazine—A case in point. Am. J. Orthopsychiatry 46:477–495.

Mason, B. G., and Menolascino, F. J. 1976. The right to treatment for mentally retarded citizens: An evolving legal and scientific interface. Creighton Law Rev. 10:124–166.

Muller, C. 1972. The overmedicated society: Forces in the marketplace for medical care. Science 176:488–492.

O'Leary, K. D., Rosenbaum, A., and Hughes, P. C. 1978. Fluorescent lighting: A purported source of hyperactive behavior. J. Abnorm. Child Psychol. 6:285–289.

Ott, J. N. 1976. Influence of fluorescent lights on hyperactivity and learning disabilities. J. Learn. Disabil. 9:22–27.

Parkin, J. M., and Fraser, M. S. 1972. Poisoning as a complication of enuresis. Dev. Med. Child Neurol. 14:727–730.

Pepper, D. 1974. Dr. Pepper reports. I. F. Stone Weekly, Feb. 18:4–5.

Renshaw, D. C. 1974. The Hyperactive Child. Nelson-Hall, Chicago.

Ross, D. M., and Ross, S. A. 1976. Hyperactivity: Research, Theory and Action. John Wiley & Sons, Inc., New York.

Safer, D. J., and Allen, R. P. 1976. Hyperactive Children: Diagnosis and Management. University Park Press, Baltimore.

Schrag, P., and Divoky, D. 1975. The Myth of the Hyperactive Child. Pantheon Books, New York.

Scott, T. J. 1970. The use of music to reduce hyperactivity in children. Am. J. Orthopsychiatry 40:677–680.

Sprague, R. L. 1973. Recommended performance measures for psychotropic drug investigations. Pharmacotherapy of Children. Special Issue of Psychopharmacology Bulletin, 85–88.

Sprague, R. L. 1977. Psychopharmacotherapy in children. In M. F. McMillan and S. Henao (eds.), Child Psychiatry: Treatment and Research. Brunner/Mazel, New York.

Sprague, R. L. 1978. Principles of clinical trials and social, ethical and legal issues of drug use in children. In J. S. Werry (ed.), Pediatric Psychopharmacology-The Use of Behavior Modifying Drugs in Children. Brunner/Mazel, New York.

Sprague, R. L., and Baxley, G. B. 1978. Drugs for behavior management, with comments on some legal aspects. In J. Wortis (ed.), Mental Retardation, Vol. 10. Brunner/Mazel, New York.

Sprague, R. L., and Gadow, K. 1977. The role of the teacher in drug treatment. In J. J. Bosco and S. S. Robin (eds.), The Hyperactive Child and Stimulant Drugs. University of Chicago Press, Chicago.

Sprague, R. L., and Sleator, E. K. 1977. Methylphenidate in hyperkinetic children: Differences in dose effects on learning and social behavior. Science 198:1274–1276.

Sprague, R. L., and Werry, J. S. 1971. Methodology of psychopharmacological studies with the retarded. In N. R. Ellis (ed.), International Review of Research in Mental Retardation, Vol 5. Academic Press, New York.

Sprague, R. L., and Werry, J. S. 1974. Psychotropic drugs and handicapped children. In L. Mahn and D. A. Sabatino (eds.), The Second Review of Special Education. JSE Press, Philadelphia.

Stewart, M. A. 1975. Treatment of bedwetting. J.A.M.A. 232:281–283.

Stewart, M. A., and Olds, S. W. 1973. Raising a Hyperactive Child. Harper, New York.

Vincent, J. P., Williams, B. J., and Elrod, T. 1977. Ratings and observations (hyperactivity by the multitrait-multimethod analyses. In R. Halliday (chair), The hyperactive child: Fact, fiction and fantasy. Symposium presented at the meeting of the American Psychological Association, August, San Francisco.

Wender, P. H. 1971. Minimal Brain Dysfunction in Children. John Wiley & Sons, Inc., New York.

Wender, P. H. 1973. The Hyperactive Child. Crown, New York.

Werry, J. S. 1978a. Measures in pediatric psychopharmacology. In J. S. Werry (ed.), Pediatric Psychopharmacology—The Use of Behavior Modifying Drugs in Children. Brunner/Mazel, New York.

Werry, J. S. (ed.) 1978b. Pediatric Psychopharmacology—The Use of Behavior Modifying Drugs in Children. Brunner/Mazel, New York.

Winchell, C. A. 1975. The Hyperkinetic Child: A Bibliography of Medical, Educational, and Behavioral Studies. Greenwood Press, Westport, Conn.

Index